Understanding the
ICD-10
Classification of
Mental Disorders

Pocket Reference

N Sartorius

SCIENCE PRESS

© 1995 Science Press Limited, 34–42 Cleveland Street, London W1P 6LB, UK.

http://www.current-science-group.com/

First published in 1995
Reprinted in 1999

British Library Cataloguing-in-Publication Data.
A catalogue record for this book is available from the British Library.

ISBN 1-85873-032-5

This book represents the findings of its author and is not necessarily the opinion of Eli Lilly and Company Ltd.

Although every effort has been made to ensure that drug doses and other information are presented accurately in this publication, the ultimate responsibility rests with the prescribing physician. Neither the publisher nor the author can be held responsible for errors or for any consequences rising from the use of information contained herein. Any product mentioned in this publication should be used in accordance with the prescribing information prepared by the manufacturers. No claims or endorsements are made for any drug or compound at present under clinical investigation.

Editor: Sarah Findlay
Designer: Claire Huntley
Typesetter: Simon Banister
Production controller: David Forrest
Printed in UK.

TABLE OF CONTENTS

INTRODUCTION

ICD-10 is an abbreviation used to describe the 10th Revision of the International Statistical Classification of Diseases and Related Health Problems. The book containing it was published in 1992, nearly 150 years after the first International Statistical Congress held in Brussels in 1853 asked William Farr — the first medical statistician of the General Register Office of England and Wales — and Marc d' Espine of Geneva in Switzerland to prepare "a uniform nomenclature of causes of death applicable in all the countries". Two years later, in Paris, during the second Statistical Congress, Farr submitted a classification in which all diseases were divided into five groups — epidemic diseases, constitutional diseases, local diseases (arranged according to their anatomical site), developmental diseases and diseases that are a direct consequence of violence. D'Espine selected a different approach: his classification was based on the nature of diseases (e.g. haematic diseases). After considerable discussion the Congress adopted a compromise list of 138 categories. Some 10 years later the classification was revised using Farr's principles, and further revisions followed in 1874, 1880 and 1886.

A few years later the International Statistical Institute, which replaced the International Statistical Congress, requested that a committee prepare a comprehensive classification of causes of death. The committee — chaired by J. Bertillon, a grandson of Achille Guillard who had introduced the resolution asking Farr and d'Espine to prepare a uniform classification — produced a proposal for such a classification that was adopted by the Institute in 1893. The classification divided diseases into generalized diseases and those localized in a particular organ or anatomical site. It was based on a classification that Bertillon, at the time the Chef de Travaux Statistiques de la Ville de Paris, used in Paris and represented a synthesis of the English, German and Swiss classifications.

Several countries adopted the Bertillon Classification of Causes of Death, and when Bertillon reported on the progress of the Classification at the International Statistical Institute meeting in

1899, the Institute expressed its pleasure and adopted a resolution recommending the use of the Classification to all statistical offices which had not yet adopted it. A year later, in Paris, the French Government organized the first International Conference for the revision of the classification of causes of death. The conference adopted Bertillon's classification and recommended that it should be revised every ten years. The French government in fact convened subsequent conferences in 1909, 1920, 1929 and 1938. The proposals for the 1929 and 1938 revisions of the International List of Causes of Death were drafted by a mixed commission composed of representatives of the International Statistical Institute and the Health Organization of the League of Nations. The subsequent revisions were all produced by international effort.

The International Health Conference, held in New York in 1946, requested that the interim commission of the World Health Organization (WHO) prepare the next revision of the International List of Causes of Death and establish an International list of Causes of Morbidity. In 1948, the government of France convened the next meeting, the International Conference for the Sixth Revision of the International List of Diseases and Causes of Death jointly with the WHO. The work on the international classification of diseases was from then on supported by national committees on vital and health statistics and carried out by the WHO, whose constitution includes the development of the classification as one of the Organization's functions. The seventh revision conference was still held in Paris: the eighth, ninth and 10th revision conferences were held in Geneva, Switzerland in 1965, 1975 and 1989. The 10th revision [1] was produced and presented after an interval longer than ten years: the development of complex health information systems and a variety of other reasons made it necessary to allow more time between the revisions. It is therefore likely that the 11th revision will not be proposed until the first decade of the next century at the earliest: in view of this, the 10th revision is constructed in a way that allows smaller changes, without a drastic overhaul of the classification as a whole.

The 1975 revision conference was significant because it adopted a number of far-reaching innovations of the ICD. It was during this conference that several additional documents — the beginning of the ICD 'family' of classifications — were presented to the delegates. These included a classification of procedures in medicine (published as a supplement to the ninth revision) and a classification of impairments and handicaps that was to be published, also as a supplement to the ninth revision, for trial purposes. The conference also marked the beginning of the production of adaptations of the ICD for specialist purposes (e.g. the development of the adaptation of the ICD for oncology, the ICD-O) and produced a series of recommendations and rules concerning matters such as lay reporting of diseases, mortality coding rules and the selection of a single cause for statistics of mortality.

Another innovation in the ninth revision was the introduction of two codes for diagnostic descriptions that contain information about the manifestation of the illness and about the underlying disease process. The convention was that a dagger (†) marked the underlying disease and an asterisk (*) the manifestation. Thus, for example, tuberculous meningitis is coded in the chapter of infectious diseases with a dagger and in the chapter dealing with nervous diseases with an asterisk. This convention is also retained in the 10th revision of the ICD. It affects several codings in the chapter dealing with mental disorders: thus, for example, dementia is coded with an asterisk in the chapter dealing with mental disorders and with a dagger in the chapter dealing with diseases of the nervous system. The categories marked with a dagger are used for reporting mortality statistics: thus, for mortality statistics all cases of tuberculosis would be counted together, while for morbidity statistics tuberculous meningitis could be reported with other forms of meningitis.

A particularly important event for the field of psychiatry was the decision of the 1975 Conference to incorporate brief descriptions of the categories included in Chapter V (mental disorders) in the ninth revision of the ICD. No other chapter has been allowed the introduction of such a glossary. Significantly, the ICD manual stated that the glossary descriptions were not intended to help the lay coder; rather, they were to assist the person making the diagnosis. The brief descriptions of the categories included in this chapter had been produced in time for the eighth revision but had to be published separately [2]. The decision to include them into the main body of the ICD has been very useful and has stimulated work on the definitions, criteria and rules concerning the classification of mental disorders.

 The 10th revision of the ICD

The 10th revision of the ICD was adopted in 1989 by the revision conference held in Geneva, and submitted to the World Health Assembly the following year. The ICD-10 was different from its predecessors in several aspects. First, the ICD-10 is constructed using an alpha-numeric coding scheme of one letter followed by three numbers (at the four character level). This innovation had the effect of more than doubling the number of categories and allowing most of the major groups of disorders to have a separate chapter. Of the 26 available letters in the English alphabet 25 have been used, each with 100 three-character categories: one letter (U) has been reserved for changes that may be necessary between revisions. In some instances the same group of diseases occupies more than one letter, for example infectious diseases span A00 to B99. The larger number of categories also allowed a more logical arrangement of disease groups and the creation of a reserve of categories within each major chapter for future expansions and revisions.

Two chapters that were considered supplementary in the ICD-9 were incorporated into the ICD-10 as ordinary chapters — the classification of external causes of injury and the classification of factors influencing health status and contact with health services. The latter decision made it easier to create the third axis for the multiaxial presentation of the ICD-10 for use in psychiatry by providing together (in Chapter XXI) all the categories for coding of contextual factors that influence the occurrence, course and outcome of mental disorders. Several of the chapters that previously contained more than one group of disorders were divided into separate chapters or rearranged: thus, for example, the chapter on the diseases of the nervous system and the sense organs has been split so that the diseases of the nervous system have a separate chapter in the 10th revision.

Another innovation in the process of preparations of the proposals for the 10th revision has been the introduction of field tests for all chapters in which a major change was foreseen. This has been done for the chapters dealing with mental and behavioural disorders, for the chapter dealing with injuries and poisoning and for the chapter dealing with external causes of morbidity and mortality.

The asterisk and dagger system introduced in the ninth revision has been modified and retained in the 10th revision for some 80 categories. A number of smaller modifications have also been undertaken to facilitate the use of the classification. For the same reason the order of chapters has been modified as little as possible from the ICD-9.

In the ninth revision the four-digit titles had often been formulated so they could not stand alone: it was usually necessary to refer to the three-digit title to determine the meaning of the category. This has been changed in the 10th revision, where every effort has been made to ensure that the four-digit categories have a title that describes the group of conditions in full and can stand alone.

 The ICD-10 family of classifications

Undoubtedly the most interesting difference between the ICD-10 and the preceding revisions was the introduction of the concept of the ICD family of classifications.

The central part of the family is the **ICD-10 three-character core classification**, which covers in its 21 chapters all diagnoses, symptoms and abnormal laboratory findings, as well as external causes of morbidity and mortality and factors influencing health status and contacts with health services.

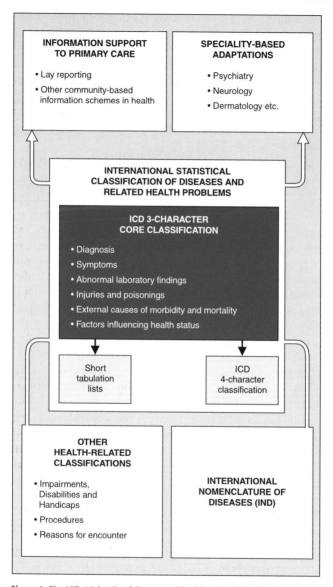

Figure 1. The ICD-10 family of disease and health-related classifications. Reproduced with permission, WHO [1].

From that core list, short tabulation lists have been developed for various purposes (e.g. hospital admission records). The three-character codes are usually subdivided, thus producing the **four-character classification**. The three- and four-character classifications are central to international communication; for this reason the revision conference recommended that no changes should be made to the content of these categories in the preparation of translations and adaptations of the ICD.

The other members of the ICD-10 family are described overleaf. Although dealing with very different topics they all have in common that their production depended on collaboration with a variety of specialists who had previously not been regularly involved in the production of the International Classification of Diseases. The development of the ICD required collaboration with lexicographers and historians of medicine; the specialty-based adaptations relied heavily on collaboration with non-governmental organizations. The development of a system for reporting from primary health care would be difficult without the participation of primary health care workers, information system specialists and mid-level health care managers. The classification of impairments, disabilities and handicaps relied on collaboration with experts from the insurance agencies, with those employed in the social sector, those dealing with rehabilitation, and others in both the governmental and nongovernmental organizations. The classification of reasons for encounter with health services should remain an important area of enquiry for health service researchers as well as for those developing the ICD. The classification of procedures in medicine also required collaboration with those involved in economic evaluation of health care and in developing standards for quality assurance in health care.

The main purpose of the **International Nomenclature of Diseases (IND)** is to provide a single recommended name for every disease entity. The production of the Nomenclature was a task that the WHO shared with the Council for International

Organizations of Medical Sciences. Several volumes of the Nomenclature have already been published; others are in preparation. The volume containing names for psychiatric diseases has not yet been produced.

A number of **specialty-based adaptations** are being produced. An adaptation of the ICD for neurological purposes (ICD-9 NA) has been prepared for the ICD-9 [3] and the same was done for the ICD-10 [4]. The adaptations make detailed provision for the recording of information likely to be useful in research and for specialized services.

Development of primary health care has been a central concern of the WHO. It was therefore logical that the Organization should undertake work on the production of a system of reporting from primary health care services that could be used in the conditions that usually prevail in developing countries. The classification of mental health problems for use in primary health care may become part of this reporting system (see pages 50–55).

The **International Classification of Impairments, Disabilities and Handicaps (ICIDH)** [5] is a particularly important member of the ICD family. Current estimates indicate that as much as 10% of the world's population has some form of disability and it is likely that the prevalence of disability will increase. Appropriate reporting of the numbers of disabled people, the impairments that have led to their disabilities and the handicaps that society imposes on those with a disability are important for the planning and evaluation of services that are established to help the disabled and their communities. The ICIDH has already proved to be a convenient tool for work in the field of rehabilitation and disability prevention. The second revision of the ICIDH, which may be submitted to the World Health Assembly for approval in 1998, will be based on results of field tests and will most probably be particularly helpful for work in the field of mental health.

The remaining members of the ICD family are also important for psychiatrists and national mental health programmes.

Mental health problems are often the main reason for consultation at different levels of health care but remain unrecognized and therefore inadequately treated. A better **classification of reasons for encounter with health services** may help in estimating the size of the mental health burden and eventually lead to better training programmes for health care workers. The **classification of procedures** used in medicine has, until recently, been of less importance for psychiatry than for other medical disciplines. The increasing use of sophisticated diagnostic procedures in psychiatry and the recognition of the high levels of co-morbidity between mental and physical disorders will bring change in this respect and render the classification of procedures in medicine just as interesting for psychiatric services as it is for services provided by other disciplines.

Chapter 1

DEVELOPMENT AND CHARACTERISTICS OF THE ICD-10 CLASSIFICATION OF MENTAL DISORDERS

 Contents of the ICD-10

The core classification of the ICD family has 21 chapters dealing with diseases as follows:

I   Certain infections and parasitic diseases (A00–B99)

II   Neoplasms (C00–D48)

III   Diseases of the blood and blood-forming organs and certain disorders involving the immune mechanism (D50–D89)

IV   Endocrine, nutritional and metabolic diseases (E00–E90)

V   Mental and behavioural disorders (F00–F99)

VI   Diseases of the nervous system (G00–G99)

VII   Diseases of the eye and adnexa (H00–H59)

VIII   Diseases of the ear and mastoid process (H60–H95)

IX   Diseases of the circulatory system (I00–I99)

X   Diseases of the respiratory system (J00–J99)

XI   Diseases of the digestive system (K00–K93)

XII   Diseases of the skin and subcutaneous system (L00–L93)

XIII   Diseases of the musculoskeletal system and connective tissue (M00–M99)

XIV   Diseases of the genitourinary system (N00–N99)

XV   Pregnancy, childbirth and the puerperium (O00–O99)

XVI   Certain conditions originating in the perinatal period (P00–P96)

XVII   Congenital malformations, deformations and chromosomal abnormalities (Q00–Q99)

XVIII   Symptoms, signs and abnormal clinical and laboratory findings, not elsewhere classified (R00–R99)

XIX   Injury, poisoning and certain other consequences of external causes (S00–T98)

XX   External causes of morbidity and mortality (V01–Y98)

XXI   Factors influencing health status and contact with health services (Z00–Z99).

Chapter V(F) is reserved for mental and behavioural disorders and chapter VI(G) deals with neurological diseases. Psychiatric practice and reporting requires the use of categories from these two chapters as well as categories from other chapters describing diseases (e.g. infectious diseases and brain tumours). In addition, reporting from psychiatric practice will frequently require coding of disorders which have no causal connection with the mental disorders (e.g. those describing co-existing physical diseases) and the use of chapters dealing with the classification of causes of suicide and accidents. Information obtained through the exploration of data reported in chapters dealing with consequences of external lesions (e.g. intoxicants), and those dealing with symptoms (e.g. hallucinations, amnesia) are also frequently of interest for psychiatry, as are those dealing with factors which influence contact with health services (e.g. pregnancy out of wedlock, unemployment).

As mentioned before, the chapter of the ICD-10 dealing with mental disorders (chapter V(F)) is the only one containing brief glossary notes about the contents of the categories (Figure 2). These glossary notes have been particularly carefully worded and every effort has been made to ensure that the formulations are fully acceptable to nongovernmental organizations and others active in the field of classification. The glossary notes were already included in the text of the ICD-9, and they have been kept similar to the earlier definitions wherever possible.

F00* **Dementia in Alzheimer's Disease (G30.-†)**

Alzheimer's disease is a primary degenerative cerebral disease of unknown etiology with characteristic neuropathological and neurochemical features. The disorder is usually insidious in onset and develops slowly but steadily over a period of several years.

F00.0* **Dementia in Alzheimer's disease with early onset (G30.0†)**

Dementia in Alzheimer's disease with onset before the age of 65, with a relatively rapid deteriorating course and with marked multiple disorders of the higher cortical functions.

Alzheimer's disease, type 2

Presenile dementia, Alzheimer's type

Primary degenerative dementia of the Alzheimer's type, presenile onset

Figure 2. Sample from short glossary. Reproduced with permission, WHO [1].

Requirements for an international classification of diseases

The ICD chapter dealing with mental disorders had to be constructed paying attention to the constraints arising in the development of any international classification as well as to constraints specific to the classification of psychiatric disorders.

1. Such a classification, if it is to be useful and used, must be based on points of agreement among health professionals, and between them and other users of the classification. The large number of professions involved in mental health care makes this requirement particularly difficult to satisfy.

2. It must be sufficiently simple to allow its easy use by all concerned. The technical language of psychiatry has always been complex and marked by conceptual differences between psychiatric schools of thought. The simplification of terms is, therefore, particularly difficult in the field of mental health.

3. The ICD must at all times aim to link classifications in existence. Thus, it must not aim to oust, compete with, or replace regional or local classifications, which often have valuable functions and are likely to be well adjusted to the situation in which they have come into existence.

4. It must be constructed in a way that will allow translations of national or special-purpose classifications into the international reference classification.

5. It must be rather conservative and theoretically unenterprising so as to remain attractive or at least acceptable to a wide variety of people of different orientations and knowledge.

6. It must be stable, and abide by the rule that changes can be introduced only when sufficient scientific data have become available to support the change and facilitate its acceptance.

7. It must take into account languages into which or from which the classification will be translated.

8. It must preserve a certain amount of continuity between successive revisions, for economic and scientific reasons.

Development of the classification of mental and behavioural disorders

The classification of mental disorders included in the ICD has been developed through a complex process lasting nearly three decades. In 1957 Professor Stengel was invited by the WHO to review the situation concerning psychiatric classifications. His report, now a classic paper in the field [6], indicated that there is little agreement among psychiatrists about the best way of classifying mental disorders; that representatives of different schools of psychiatry vigorously defend the classification that their school of thought has produced, regardless of the lack of validating evidence; and that new classifications were being produced by many different schools of psychiatry. A few years later the WHO started its programme of epidemiology of mental disorders, in which work on the standardization of psychiatric diagnosis, classification and statistics (Programme A), had been given highest priority [7,8]. Programme A relied on a nuclear group composed of leading psychiatrists and statisticians from a variety of countries who met annually in different parts of the world, each time with a large group of psychiatrists from the host country and neighbouring countries. Discussion centred on major groups of psychiatric disorders, taking them on in turn. At each meeting a series of cases was presented, either live, recorded on film or video, or described in a narrative. The differences in diagnostic assessments of these cases served as a point of departure for discussions about ways of structuring a classification that would minimize the probability of disagreement. A series of publications, the glossary of categories included in the ICD-8, methodological guidelines for the exploration of diagnosis and a detailed proposal for the ICD-8 were among the results of Programme A. More importantly, the programme has created an atmosphere of interest in matters of diagnosis and classification and created a worldwide network of individuals and centres willing to continue collaborating on these matters.

In another part of the WHO programme of epidemiological psychiatry [9], the emphasis was on the production of instruments for a standardized examination of patients and their characteristics. The results of these efforts were useful to further work on diagnosis and classification as well.

In 1980, the WHO, in collaboration with the Alcohol, Drug Abuse and Mental Health Administration (ADAMHA), undertook an even more ambitious project aiming to further improve diagnostic tools, the classification of mental disorders and epidemiological reporting about mental illness and about factors relevant to its occurrence, course and outcome. Numerous studies and small scale meetings of experts organized in the framework of the Joint Project prepared the ground for a major conference on Psychiatric Diagnosis and Classification in Copenhagen [10].The conference brought together leaders of psychiatry, behavioural science, public health and statistics from countries all over the world. The review of the work undertaken over the past two decades led to recommendations which became the basis for the next 15 years of work which the WHO and ADAMHA undertook jointly [11]. One result of this project was the proposal for the 10th revision of the ICD; another, the instruments (e.g. the SCAN — Schedule for Comprehensive Assessment in Neuropsychiatry; and the CIDI — Comprehensive International Diagnostic Interview) for the assessment of characteristics of the patient, applicable and tested in different cultural settings.

 ## Characteristics of the ICD-10 classification of mental disorders

The classification of mental disorders in the ICD-10 has certain characteristics which make it unique.

- The classification is based on consensus among psychiatrists and other mental health workers belonging to widely different schools of thought and working in very different conditions. In the preparation of the proposals for the classification the WHO has consulted experts in more than 60 countries, sent them drafts of the texts of criteria and other materials for review and requested their views and guidance. Nongovernmental organizations were invited to participate in this process as well as national organizations and groups interested in the development of classifications. The American Psychiatric Association (APA) — which has made a major contribution to the development of psychiatric classifications by developing the third revision of its Diagnostic and Statistical Manual (DSM-III) — has collaborated in the preparation of the ICD-10 under the auspices of ADAMHA, provided excellent contributions to the ICD-10 and made a major effort to make the fourth revision of the DSM (DSM-IV) almost fully compatible with the ICD-10. Collaboration with other national groups such as the experts who developed the French classification of mental disorders in childhood has also been maintained, and resulted in arrangements which allow the translation of codes between classifications. Governments have also been consulted in a regular manner, as have professional groups dealing with special problems such as sleep disorders.

- The ICD-10 classification of mental health disorders (ICD-10 MNH) has been produced in several versions for different groups of users and for use in specific situations. The decision to create different versions of the classification introduced the need to consult and involve groups which have not worked on psychiatric classifications in the past, such as general practitioners. These contacts have been most productive and helped in making the classification acceptable to its users. The various versions of the ICD-10 classification of mental disorders are described below. They are fully compatible with each other and with other relevant parts of the ICD (e.g. with the classification of factors influencing encounters with health services).

- The ICD-10 MNH has been developed taking into account not only the findings of the extensive review of the literature in various languages carried out during the preparation of the proposals for the classification, but also the results of field tests of the ICD-10 versions. Experts and institutions in 40 countries have participated in these trials, which were carried out to establish the usefulness of the classification. Case descriptions, video-taped and live interviews with patients were the source of materials for the tests, which were carried out in routine clinical and research conditions in the languages of the various countries participating in the trials. The trials established that the classification was easy to use in the different countries, that psychiatrists using it can reach agreement in their diagnostic assignments and that the classification adequately covered the needs of psychiatrists and others dealing with the diagnosis and treatment of patients with mental disorders [12]. Numerous publications describing the results of these trials in different language areas have appeared already and others are in preparation.

- The ICD-10 MNH has been developed simultaneously in different languages, unlike previous revisions of the ICD. The texts produced in English were translated into French, Spanish, Chinese, Italian, German, Portuguese, Japanese, Korean and other languages while the material was still in draft. Wherever difficulties of translation were discovered the originals in English were adjusted, thus allowing the development of equivalent versions of the texts in different languages rather than producing translations from a single source language into all the others. The ICD-10 Clinical Descriptions and Diagnostic Guidelines (CDDG) [13] version is now available in 22 languages; the Diagnostic Criteria for Research (DCR) [14] in 10, and the Primary Health Care (PHC) version has been tested in a variety of languages and will be published in those languages in the very near future.

- The classification is accompanied by a variety of materials which facilitate its use. These materials include:

  (i) lexical descriptions of terms used in the description of categories [15–17];

  (ii) research instruments allowing a computerized assignment of cases assessed by them to diagnostic categories [18–20];

  (iii) symptom checklists [21]; and

  (iv) conversion tables allowing a translation of ICD-10 terms into terms and categories used in the ninth and eighth revisions of the ICD.

- The classification has been developed in close collaboration with a number of centres of excellence. These centres coordinated the field trials, translated the texts into major world languages, helped in the production of training materials and in the conduct of training courses necessary to ensure the proper use of the classification and in numerous other tasks linked to the programme. The centres did not cease their function with the publication of the ICD: on the contrary, their function of assisting users, carrying out research, recording experiences with the ICD and so forth has gained amplitude and strength. The centres are each responsible for work in a number of countries which usually share traditions in psychiatry and language use. They are in located in Aarhus (Denmark), Beijing and Shanghai (China), Bangalore (India), Cairo (Egypt), Campinas (Brazil), Lübeck (Germany), Luxembourg (Luxembourg), Madrid (Spain), Moscow (Russia), Nagasaki (Japan), Naples (Italy), Oxford (UK), Rockville (USA) and Wellington (New Zealand) (Figure 3).

- A guiding principle of the ICD-10 classification of mental disorders was that the needs of practice of work with mentally ill people, worldwide, have to be taken into account as much as scientific requirements and public health needs. This has led to (1) the decision to include categories for diagnoses which are frequently used in some countries but whose nosological status is still uncertain (e.g. mixed anxiety and depression; brief recurrent depression; neurasthenia); (2) the significant expansion of the parts of the classification dealing with acute psychotic disorders frequently seen in developing countries; (3) the decision to avoid taking social functioning as a diagnostic indicator, since the normal social functioning is so different in different sociocultural settings that its use in an international classification could lead to disagreement and misunderstanding; (4) the inclusion of categories which serve to accommodate relatively recently introduced diagnoses describing conditions of potentially great public health interest (e.g. mild cognitive disorder); and (5) the formulation of criteria in the clinical guidelines in terms easy to use by the practising psychiatrist. Thus, for example, words such as `usually' or `very often' have been used in describing particular syndromes whenever it appeared that a rigidly stated requirement could be difficult to use for a clinician.

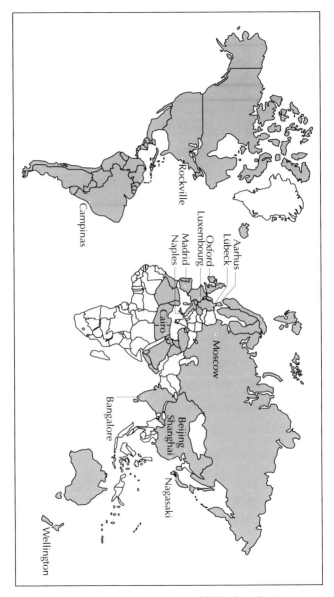

Figure 3. WHO reference and training centres and field trial coordinating centres.

Chapter 2

INNOVATIONS IN THE ICD-10 CLASSIFICATION OF MENTAL DISORDERS

A number of innovations have been introduced in the ICD-10. These include:

(1) A change of the manner in which disorders due to abuse of alcohol and other drugs are categorized (Figure 4). While in the previous revisions alcohol and drug problems were first categorized by the clinical syndrome which was present at the time of examination, the 10th revision of the ICD provides a code at the three character level for the drug of abuse, to be followed on the fourth character place by the code for the syndrome which the abuse of the substance has produced. This makes it easier to estimate the total size of the public health problem due to the abuse of a particular substance. It also facilitates reporting on patients who, in the course of their illness, show different clinical manifestations related to the use of the same substance.

(2) Several additions were made to the group of codes dealing with schizophrenic disorders (e.g. the schizotypal disorder and the postschizophrenic depression). The group of acute psychotic states has been separated from schizophrenia (Figure 5). Clinical traditions in a number of countries and a number of studies seem to indicate that the schizophrenias are a group of disorders different from the more transient psychotic states variously labelled with such terms as `bouffee delirante', `psychogenic psychosis', `cycloid psychosis' and `brief reactive psychosis'. Opinions differ about whether typical schizophrenic symptoms can be found in these disorders and whether stress is a necessary trigger or precipitant of these disorders. Most of these disorders are of relatively short duration and may have an excellent prognosis; it was therefore felt that it would be important to provide a three-character category with a title that is less loaded and stigmatized than schizophrenia and to carry out further research into the nature and outcome of these dis-

ICD-9	ICD-10
Alcoholic Psychoses (291)	*Mental and behavioral disorders*
Delirium tremens	*due to use of*
Korsakov's psychosis	F10 Alcohol
Other alcoholic dementia	F11 Opioids
Other alcoholic hallucinations	F12 Cannabinoids
Pathological drunkeness	F13 Sedatives and hypnotics
Alcoholic jealousy	F14 Cocaine
	F15 Other stimulants
Drug Psychoses (292)	F16 Hallucinogens
Drug withdrawal	F17 Tobacco
Paranoid and hallucinatory	F18 Volatile solvents
states induced by drugs	F19 Other/multiple substances
Pathological drug intoxication	
	Code synrome for each
Alcohol dependence syndrome	*category as*
(303)	.0 Intoxication
	.2 Harmful use
Drug dependence (304)	.3 Withdrawal state
Morphine	.4 Withdrawal with delirium
Barbiturate	.5 Psychotic disorder
Cocaine	.6 Amnesiac disorder
Cannabis	.7 Residual and late onset
Amphetamine	psychotic
Hallucinogen	.8 Other
Combinations	.9 Unspecified
Nondependent abuse of drugs	
(305)	

Alcohol	Barbiturate
Tobacco	Morphine
Cannabis	Cocaine
Hallucinogen	Amphetamine
Antidepressant	Other

Figure 4. A comparison of the ICD-9 and ICD-10 classifications of disorders due to substance abuse. Reproduced with permission, WHO [1,2].

orders. The advantage of this arrangement is that a diagnosis can be made without consideration of the course of the disorder. The disadvantage may be that a change of diagnostic label

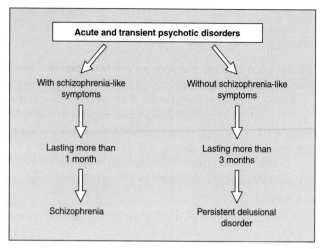

Figure 5. Scheme for the ICD-10 classification of acute and transient psychotic disorders, schizophrenia and persistent delusional disorder.

may be necessary if the disorder persists. It was felt that this way of proceeding is preferable, particularly in developing countries in which there are many patients who are admitted with acute psychotic symptoms that disappear after a few weeks. The time criterion for acute and transient psychotic disorders which also have symptoms of schizophrenia is different from that used for disorders which do not show any schizophrenia-like symptoms.

The adoption of the one-month limit for the diagnosis of schizophrenia has also been motivated by the necessity to reject the notion that schizophrenia is a chronic and long-lasting disorder in each case. The WHO studies of schizophrenia in different cultures [22,23] demonstrated that in all cultures there are patients who had typically schizophrenic symptoms and whose illness had subsided in less than six months from the onset of the disorder. It therefore seemed more logical to remove the requirement for chronicity from the definition and assume that the term schizophrenia describes a syndrome with a variety of causes and a variety of outcomes depending on a mixture of genetic, physical, social and cultural influences.

The distinction of acute and transient psychotic disorders from other psychotic disorders such as schizophrenia also required definitions of *acute* and abrupt onset and the introduction of the notion of a `polymorphic' clinical picture referring to a rapidly changing state in which a variety of psychotic symptoms make their appearance and last for only a short time. It was hoped that the definition of these terms would find general acceptance and be used in studies examining the development and course of psychotic and other disorders.

The diagnosis *simple schizophrenia* has been a point of controversy over the past several decades. It was decided to retain it in the 10th revision of the ICD because of its continued use in a number of countries and because of the need to study further the relationship of this condition with schizotypal disorders and the schizoid personality disorder. The schizophrenia categories also include the category *postschizophrenic depression,* referring to a depressive episode arising in the aftermath of a schizophrenic illness. The depressive episodes which are coded here may be due to depression, neuroleptic medication or the impaired volition and affective changes occurring as part of the schizophrenic illness itself; in the absence of good evidence about these episodes, which are described in as many as 10% of all patients treated with neuroleptic drugs, it seemed important to provide a category that will facilitate future studies of these states.

(3) Behavioural syndromes associated with physiological dysfunction and hormonal change have been brought together and organized in a more meaningful manner, and the classification of this group of disorders has been expanded to correspond to new knowledge about these disorders and the growing needs of general hospital and liaison psychiatry.

(4) The categories dealing with affective disorders have also been changed. The classification of depressive states has been rearranged and the categories dealing with depression, mania,

and bipolar disorder have been brought into proximity with persistent affective disorders (e.g. dysthymia). A new category has been added for the coding of recurrent brief depressive disorder. This category serves to accommodate depressive states which satisfy the symptomatic criteria for depression but not the duration criteria. As is the case with other conditions of unclear nosological status the provision of a category will make it possible to accumulate more evidence about the condition, thus facilitating the decision about the best way of classifying it.

Another category which has been added to the classification is reserved for *mixed anxiety and depressive disorder,* a condition that is frequently seen in psychiatric outpatient practice and in general medical services. This category, and several others such as the category of *adjustment disorders,* are likely to be used more frequently in primary health care and their inclusion into the classification is also a reflection of the growing recognition of the fact that a large proportion of patients contacting general health services suffer from psychological problems, among which are many that are not easily classifiable in classification systems made by psychiatrists on the basis of their experience in psychiatric practice.

(5) After considerable consultation with psychiatrists in different countries it was decided to retain the category of *neurasthenia* in the classification. The diagnosis is still regularly used in a number of countries and a place for coding of that diagnosis therefore has to be provided. In addition, and more importantly, several studies have shown that when also studied with standardized research instruments, a significant proportion of cases given the clinical diagnosis of neurasthenia cannot be classified into any other category. The current emergence of interest in the syndromes characterized by excessive fatigue and fatiguability also justifies the provision of categories which will allow the separate coding of neurasthenia.

(6) *Culture-specific disorders* is a term used to describe conditions which appear more frequently in one culture than in others. According to their characteristics, many of these disorders can be classified in a category of the international

classification. However, there are also conditions which are difficult to classify and about which we need to learn more before we can decide how best to place them. The fact that many of them are transient and rich in symptoms, and that some of them appear in areas in which there are few mental health specialists and poor routine statistical systems in operation makes their study more difficult. A lexicon of terms frequently used in transcultural research, including a number of terms used to describe such culture-specific syndromes, is in preparation and will be published in the near future: meanwhile, an appendix has been added to the DCR publication [14] containing the description of 12 such syndromes:

Amok (a syndrome described in particular in Indonesia and Malaysia)

Dhat, dhatu, jiryan, shen k'uei, shen kui (India and China)

Koro, jinjin bemar, suk yeong, suo-yang (south-east Asia, south China)

Latah (Indonesia and Malaysia)

Nerfiza, nerves, nevra, nervios (Egypt, northern Europe, Greece, Mexico, south and central America)

Paleng, frigophobia (China, south-east Asia)

Pibloqtoq, Arctic Hysteria (Inuits living within Arctic circle)

Susto, espanto (Mexico, central and south America)

Taijin kyofusho, shinkeishitsu, anthropophobia (Japan)

Ufufuyane, saka (southern Africa, among Bantus and Zulus)

Uqamairineq (Inuits within the Arctic circle)

Windigo (indigenous people of northeastern North America)

In each instance a brief description of the culture-specific syndromes is followed by a suggested ICD-10 code, a list of potentially related syndromes and selected references providing information about the syndrome.

(7) New categories have also been added to the group dealing with disorders of personality (e.g. pathological gambling). A place for the coding of *borderline personality disorder* has been provided, in a subcategory of *emotionally unstable personality disorders*. As is the case with some other categories which provide for conditions whose nosological status is not

fully clarified, this category should help to accumulate evidence for decisions about the assignment of this diagnosis.

(8) A major revision has been made in that part of the classification dealing with child psychiatric disorders. The number of categories foreseen for the coding of mental disorders in childhood has been significantly expanded, reflecting the rapid development of knowledge about these disorders and their importance in public health. Ten categories are now reserved for disorders of psychological development: these include specific developmental disorders of speech and language, scholastic skills and motor function, mixed developmental disorders and pervasive developmental disorders such as autism. The syndromes of Rett and Asperger have been included as four-character categories although their nosological status has only recently been generally clarified. A `mixed' category — *Overactive disorder associated with mental retardation and stereotyped movements* (F84.4) — has also been included because of its probable practical utility. Another 10 categories have been given to disorders usually beginning in childhood and adolescence; these include hyperkinetic disorder, conduct disorder, mixed disorders of conduct and emotions, disorders of social functioning and emotional and behavioural disorders with onset usually occurring in children and adolescents. The arrangement of four-character categories has also been changed, whilst trying to maintain correspondence between the ninth and 10th revision codes wherever possible.

A glance at the four-character core classification of mental disorders in the ICD-10 (see Appendix A) will inform the reader about the categories and their arrangement; a series of comments about the various new categories is also included in the introductory parts of the CDDG [13].

 Differences between international and national classifications

In addition to the international classification there are numerous national classifications of mental disorders. Some of these are fully translatable into the international classification, others only in part. Some differ in the principles used in the organization of the classification (e.g. classifications based on psychoanalytic theory), others in the arrangements of the categories. The main conceptual differences between the international and the different national classifications can be summarized as follows:

(1) The ICD must be reflective of the way in which health services function because one of its main goals is to provide a statistical tool for the recording of information from services. Thus, if a category of unclear nosological status is frequently used, a provision must be made for its recording. Hence, a category such as mixed anxiety and depressive disorders will be included because the condition is often reported by practising physicians. National classifications, on the other hand, often represent the consensus of specialists in the field about what is allowable as a category. The national professional classification may decide that the mixed anxiety and depressive disorders are not nosologically well defined and that therefore these states cannot be classified in a specific category.

(2) The ICD aims to serve international communication as well as national reporting needs. This means that the international classification seeks to use terms and categories which will be acceptable and used in the largest possible number of settings. The makers of a national classification do not have that preoccupation unless they wish to facilitate the use of their classification outside the national borders. The planned international edition of the Diagnostic and Statistical Manual of the American Psychiatric Association (DSM-IV International Edition), for example, has been tailored in a manner that should make its use abroad easier.

(3) The ICD, once approved by various scientific and advisory bodies, has to be submitted for approval to the representatives of governments of countries which will make the use of the ICD compulsory for its health services. National classifications are approved by professional associations and, if they are to be used in the national health service, they must be accompanied by a translation into terms of the official (ICD) classification.

Changes in national classifications are therefore easier to make and when made can be more dramatic than those in an international classification which serves a large number of countries and innumerable health services.

(4) The ICD uses a single system to cover the classification of all diseases as well as other items, useful in reporting for the health services (e.g. reasons for contact with health services). The national classifications most often deal with a group of diseases (e.g. mental disorders) which are the usual reasons for intervention by a single profession (e.g. psychiatry). The disadvantage for users of national classifications is that they often have to code diagnoses of their patients using two systems, one for diagnoses belonging to their field using a national professional classification, and the second using another, different system of classification for the coding of other diseases and for reimbursement purposes.

(5) The ICD can be presented as a multiaxial classification but its construction and basic form is uniaxial (with variable axes such as location or aetiology). Some of the major national classifications, including the DSM-III and DSM-IV propose the use of a multiaxial system of classification on a routine basis, despite its relative complexity, because of its educational and pragmatic benefits.

(6) The ICD-10 classification of mental disorders has introduced the principle of multiple versions of the classification for different types of users. National classifications are usually produced in one version, not least because of the difficulty of ensuring the collaboration of other professional and service groups necessary for the production of other versions (see page 16) and because of the lesser interest that the profession has in the use of its classification by members of other professional groups (e.g. the general practitioner).

(7) The international classification is being produced in collaboration with various national and international nongovernmental organizations and relies on two networks of centres for its creation and updating. The first network is composed of the

officially designated centres dealing with all aspects of classification; the second contains the centres specifically dealing with the classification of mental and neurological disorders.

(8) The international classification has been developed taking into account the results of a broad international consultation and of field trials of the draft of the classification. Numerous countries and centres operating in different languages participated in the effort, as shown in Figure 6.

Version	Number of countries	Number of centres
Clinical guidelines	39	112
Research criteria	32	150
Primary care	26	41
Multiaxial presentation	20	65

Figure 6. Participants in the field trials of the different versions of the classification of mental disorders in accordance with ICD-10.

(9) The International Classification of Mental and Behavioural Disorders is a part of the ICD-10 and as such is already the official classification used in reporting from health services and often for quality assurance control in all member countries of the WHO that have agreed to use the ICD (the vast majority of the countries of the world). Despite its imperfections, the ICD provides the best vehicle for comparative studies and international and national investigations and comparisons. No national professional classification has similar width of application, exists in so many languages, or is likely to be as widely used.

The relationship between the ICD-10 and the DSM-IV classifications of mental disorders

The development, by the American Psychiatric Association, of the third edition of the Diagnostic and Statistical Manual (DSM-III) represented a major step forward in the development of classifications in psychiatry. In no other country was there ever such a large number of psychiatric teachers, researchers and practitioners involved in the production of a classification system, accompanied by operational definitions for each category and a variety of other materials facilitating the use of the system and justifying its arrangements. What looked impossible, or at best improbable, had in fact happened — the psychiatric profession in a country defined the field of its action by defining the conditions which it believed it could treat or prevent. The appearance of the DSM-III also gave courage to psychiatrists in other countries and opened the way to an international effort directed towards the production of an important component of a common language in psychiatry — an international classification of mental disorders defined in operational detail. The experience gained in the production of the DSM-III was invaluable in the work on the ICD-10, and frequent involvement of many American mental health workers in the production of the ICD-10 helped to avoid mistakes and gain time. The production of the DSM-IV was almost simultaneous with the production of the ICD-10, and through the effort of the ADAMHA (containing, at that time, the National Institutes of Mental Health, Alcohol and Drug Abuse) numerous consultations and working contacts between the groups working on the two classifications took place, with excellent results. One of the results of this collaboration is the close compatibility of the ICD-10 and the DSM-IV, which in its international edition will carry ICD-10 category numbers alongside its definitions of categories. The definitions of categories are also to a large extent compatible. Some differences remain, as would be expected in the light of considerations listed above and the need for national classifications to remain responsive to the specific needs prevailing in that country.

Numerous recent articles have drawn attention to the points which should be taken into account in comparing the ICD-10 with the DSM-IV [24], so that the interested reader will have no difficulty in finding additional information about the subject.

Problems of terminology

The term `neurotic' is still retained for occasional use in the ICD-10. No definition of the term has been attempted in the body of the classification and its continued presence is meant to facilitate the use of the classification for those who still use the term `neurosis'. `Psychotic' has also been retained as a convenient descriptive term, particularly in F23 — *Acute and transient psychotic disorders.* Its use does not involve assumptions about psychodynamic mechanisms, but simply indicates the presence of hallucinations, delusions or a limited number of severe abnormalities of behaviour such as gross excitement and overactivity, marked psychomotor retardation and catatonic behaviour.

The term `disorder' is used throughout the ICD-10 classification of mental disorders in order to avoid even greater problems inherent in the use of terms such as `illness' and `disease'. `Disorder' is not an exact term, but is used here to imply the existence of a clinically recognizable set of symptoms or behaviour associated in most cases with distress. Wherever possible, reference to social functioning is avoided and users are explicitly warned that social deviance or conflict alone is not a mental disorder.

The term `psychogenic' has not been used in the titles of categories, in view of its different meanings in different languages and psychiatric traditions. It still occurs occasionally in the text indicating that the diagnostician regards identifiable life events or difficulties as playing an important role in the genesis of the disorder.

The term `psychosomatic' is not used in the ICD-10 because of an earlier recommendation of a WHO expert group that the term should be avoided because its use might be taken to imply that psychological factors play no role in the occurrence, course or outcome of diseases that are not so labelled. When clinicians wish to indicate the linkage between a psychological state or factor and a somatic problem they are advised to use two codes, one for the illness (e.g. eczema) and another to indicate psychological factors (e.g. F54. *Psychological or behavioural factors associated with diseases or disorders classified elsewhere*). Some of the disorders that are labelled psychosomatic in other classifications can be accomodated under categories F45 *(somatoform disorders),* F50 *(eating disorders)* and F52 *(sexual dysfunction)*.

The terms `impairment', `disability' and `handicap' are used in the sense described in the International Classification of Impairments, Disabilities and Handicaps [25]. `Impairment' refers to the loss or abnormality of a structure or function (e.g. memory loss or loss of limb), `disability' to the restriction or impossibility to perform in social and professional roles, and `handicap' to the disadvantage which society imposes on an individual with a disability.

Numerous other terms used in the description of categories are also defined differently by the various schools of psychiatry and in different languages. The WHO has therefore produced several lexica [15–17] describing terms used in the description of categories and is about to publish a multilingual dictionary giving the best equivalent for terms used in psychiatry in English, French, German, Portuguese and Spanish. Equivalents in Arabic, Chinese, Japanese and Russian may have to be produced in separate volumes.

 The coding conventions

Each of the categories in the ICD-10 has a code composed of four characters. The first of these is a letter designating the chapter, usually a group of diseases of particular interest to a medical specialty. The second describes a subgroup of disorders, e.g. affective disorders. The third character, also a digit, describes the disease or disorder and the fourth character, a digit, gives more detail about the condition, e.g. describing its form or course. Figure 7 shows the structure of an ICD-10 code.

Further subdivisions using the sixth or seventh character place can be made for specific purposes of a study or a specialized service.

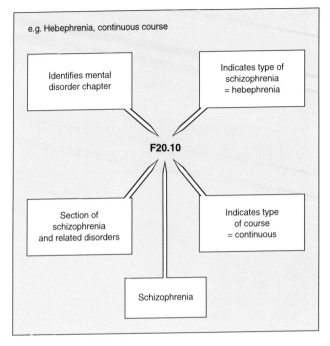

Figure 7. Structure of an ICD-10 code.

The family of the ICD-10 classification of mental disorders

The concept of a `family' of instruments and classifications which has been used in the construction of the ICD-10 system has been further expanded and developed in relation to the classification of mental and neurological disorders. This family is composed of the following members:

(a) different versions of the classifications of mental and behavioural disorders:

- the short glossary (see page 12)
- the clinical descriptions and clinical guidelines (CDDG)

- the diagnostic criteria for research (DCR)*
- the multiaxial presentation of the ICD-10 for use in: work with childhood mental disorders work with mental disorders in adults
- the primary health care classification
- the psychiatric and neurological adaptations of the ICD-10

(b) Assessment Instruments

- Composite International Diagnostic Interview (CIDI)
- Schedule for Clinical Assessment in Neuropsychiatry (SCAN)
- International Personality Disorder Examination (IPDE)
- Disability Assessment Schedule (DAS)
- Symptoms checklists and their glossaries

(c) Training materials and other materials facilitating the use of the ICD-10:

- Fascicles developed for the needs of particular groups of users (e.g. a mental retardation fascicle, a fascicle on headache and a sleep disorder fascicle)
- Lexicons — of psychiatric and mental health terms (first and second editions), of alcohol and drug abuse terms, of culture-specific terms
- A multilingual dictionary of ICD terms
- Training Materials — Casebook, Standard Curricula for workshops dealing with the ICD-10 Classification of Mental Disorders

(d) Crosswalks, for translation of codes between ICD-10 and previous revisions of the ICD (ICD-9, ICD-8).

- The following pages will describe the materials listed above.

---

*A combination of the materials from the short glossary, the CDDG and DCR versions accompanied by notes for users has also been published recently [25] (see page 75)

Chapter 3

THE CLINICAL DESCRIPTIONS AND DIAGNOSTIC GUIDELINES (CDDG VERSION)

The Clinical Descriptions and Diagnostic Guidelines (CDDG) publication [13] is central to the ICD-10 Mental Health (ICD-10 MNH) Family of Classifications and has been published in more than twenty languages (see Appendix B). The CDDG is primarily intended for use by the clinical psychiatrist. At the same time, however, it contains information which needs to be employed whenever the Diagnostic Criteria for Research (DCR) are used and when other versions of the ICD-10 MNH are examined or explained.

The CDDG contains, for each *group* of disorders, an introduction giving a brief summary of the main issues that may arise in the process of classification of the particular group of disorders. Each disorder is then listed, and a description is provided of the main clinical features and any important but less specific associated features of that disorder. This *clinical description* is followed by *diagnostic guidelines,* which indicate the number and balance of symptoms usually required in order to make a diagnosis with confidence. The guidelines are worded in a manner which allows clinicians to make a diagnosis in clinical work even when the information about a condition is not fully available or when the clinical picture is not completely clear. In some instances the diagnostic guidelines are provided for groups of disorders in addition to those which relate to individual disorders, to avoid repetition. The diagnostic guidelines are followed by notes about differential diagnosis and by a listing of inclusion and exclusion terms (i.e. diagnostic labels that should be categorized in that diagnostic category or excluded from it), as shown in Figure 8.

When the requirements laid down in the diagnostic guidelines are clearly fulfilled, the diagnosis can be regarded as `confident'. When the requirements are only partially fulfilled,

Overview of block: **F20–F29**	Table listing all the disorders covered in chapter ***F20–F29 — Schizophrenia, schizotypal and delusional disorders***
Introduction	General comments on the conditions listed in this block, e.g. schizophrenia, schizotypal disorders, delusional disorders and schizoaffective disorders

F20	Schizophrenia:
	    clinical descriptions
	    diagnostic guidelines

F20.0	Paranoid schizophrenia:
	    clinical descriptions
	    diagnostic guidelines
	    inclusion criteria
	    differential diagnosis
	    exclusion criteria

Figure 8. Layout of a CDDG chapter.

it is nevertheless useful to record a diagnosis for most purposes. It is then for the diagnostician and other users of the diagnostic statements to decide whether to record the lesser degrees of confidence (such as `provisional' if more information is to come, or `tentative' if more information is unlikely to become available) that are implied in these circumstances. Statements about the duration of symptoms in the CDDG are also intended as general guidelines rather than strict requirements; clinicians should use their own judgement about the appropriateness of making a diagnosis when the duration of particular symptoms is slightly longer or shorter than specified.

The guidelines contain more material than is necessary for assigning diagnoses into categories. The decision to produce them in this form is based on the recognition that the guidelines will be used in the teaching of psychiatry.

In addition to the description of categories, taking most of the book, there are several other chapters in the CDDG which need a mention. First, there is a list of centres which have coordinated field trials of the classification, translated the texts into their languages and participated in a particularly active way in the collection and examination of comments and suggestions made by consultants and participants in field trials (see pages xi and xii of [13]. Heads of training and reference centres can be contacted to obtain further information or to discuss ideas for studies involving the classification).

The introductory chapter provides information about the layout of the CDDG, differences between the ninth and 10th revisions of the ICD, and specific suggestions for users, for example about the way in which multiple diagnoses should be recorded. This is followed by comment on different groups of disorders included in the CDDG, indicating, for example, where new categories have been added and how the criteria were selected.

The text of the clinical description is also preceeded by a list of all categories and followed by an annex listing other conditions from the ICD-10 which are often encountered in clinical practice. This includes codes for some infectious diseases of the CNS, neoplasms of the CNS, endocrine, nutritional and metabolic diseases (e.g. iodine deficiency), a full listing of neurological disorders, some diseases of the sense organs and of the circulatory, respiratory, digestive, musculoskeletal and genitourinary systems, and of the skin. Three codes from the chapter dealing with pregnancy, childbirth and the puerperium are listed — medical abortion, maternal care for fetal abnormality (e.g. for damage from alcohol) and for maternal mental disorders classifiable elsewhere but complicating pregnancy, childbirth and the puerperium. Congenital malformations and chromosomal abnormalities relevant for psychiatry are also listed, as are symptoms and signs, intoxications and intentional self-harm, assault and adverse effects of psychotrophic drugs. The classification of factors influencing health status and contacts with health services is given in full.

The last part of the book gives a list of principal investigators who have contributed to the work on the ICD-10. These are ordered by country and represent a useful list of individuals interested and knowledgeable in matters related to the classification in different countries. An index of disorders lists all diagnostic terms and titles of categories alphabetically. A sample page of the CDDG is shown in Figure 9.

F20.0 Paranoid schizophrenia

This is the commonest type of schizophrenia in most parts of the world. The clinical picture is dominated by relatively stable, often paranoid, delusions, usually accompanied by hallucinations, particularly of the auditory variety, and perceptual disturbances. Disturbances of affect, volition, and speech, and catatonic symptoms, are not prominent.

Examples of the most common paranoid symptoms are:

(a) delusions of persecution, reference, exalted birth, special mission, bodily change, or jealousy;

(b) hallucinatory voices that threaten the patient or give commands, or auditory hallucinations without verbal form, such as whistling, humming, or laughing;

(c) hallucinations of smell or taste, or of sexual or other bodily sensations; visual hallucinations may occur but are rarely predominant.

Thought disorder may be obvious in acute states, but if so it does not prevent the typical delusions or hallucinations from being described clearly. Affect is usually less blunted than in other varieties of schizophrenia but a minor degree of incongruity is common, as are mood disturbances such as irritability, sudden anger, fearfulness, and suspicion. Negative symptoms such as blunting of affect and impaired volition are often present but do not dominate the clinical picture.

The course of paranoid schizophrenia may be episodic, with partial or complete remissions, or chronic. In chronic cases, the florid symptoms persist over years and it is difficult to distinguish discrete episodes. The onset tends to be later than in the hebephrenic and catatonic forms.

Diagnostic guidelines

The general criteria for a diagnosis of schizophrenia (see introduction to F20 above) must be satisfied. In addition, hallucinations and/or delusions must be prominent, and disturbances of affect, volition and speech, and catatonic symptoms must be relatively inconspicuous. the hallucination will usually be of the kind described in (b) and (c) above.

Continued

Delusions can be of almost any kind but delusions of control, influence, or passivity, and persecutory beliefs of various kinds are the most characteristic.

Includes: paraphrenic schizophrenia

Differential diagnosis. It is important to exclude epileptic and drug-induced psychoses, and to remember that persecutory delusions might carry little diagnostic weight in people from certain countries or cultures.

Excludes: involutional paranoid state (F22.8); paranoia (F22.0)

Figure 9. Sample page from CDDG version. Reproduced with permission, WHO [13].

Chapter 4

DIAGNOSTIC CRITERIA FOR RESEARCH (DCR VERSION)

The Diagnostic Criteria for Research (DCR) [14] are produced to help research workers in the field of psychiatry. They do not contain the descriptions of the clinical concepts upon which the research criteria are based, nor any comments on commonly associated features which may well be relevant for both clinicians and researchers; thus, the DCR should be used together with the CDDG.

The book containing the DCR is organized in a similar way to the CDDG. There are two annexes; the first provides provisional criteria for the definition of diagnostic categories whose clinical and scientific status is uncertain and about which more information would be useful. Three of these disorders are mood disorders (*seasonal affective disorder, bipolar II disorder, rapid cycling bipolar disorder*) and two concern personality disorders (*narcissistic personality disorder* and *passive–aggressive personality disorder*). The second annex describes culture-specific disorders (see pages 24–25) and will be useful in conjunction with the Lexicon of terms used in cross-cultural research (in preparation). A list of centres which have coordinated field trials is listed in Appendix C, useful for those who wish to establish collaboration with groups interested in research on matters relevant to diagnosis and classification in their geographical area or in other locations.

The section providing research criteria is central to the volume. Like other research criteria, the criteria of the DCR-10 are deliberately restrictive: their use allows the selection of groups of individuals whose symptoms resemble each other in clearly stated ways. Homogenous groups of patients are useful for certain types of research; researchers wishing to study the overlap of disorders or the best way to define boundaries between them may therefore need to supplement the criteria with provisions which allow the inclusion of `atypical cases'. The criteria in the DCR descriptions of categories are labelled with letters and/or numbers to indicate their place in a hierarchy of generality and importance. General criteria, which must be fulfilled by all members of a group of disorders (such as the general criteria for all varieties of dementia, or the main types of schizophrenia) are labelled with a capital G, plus a number. Obligatory criteria for individual disorders are by capital letters alone (A,B,...); numbers (1,2,...) and lower case letters (a,b,...) are used to identify further groups and subgroups of characteristics, of which only some are required for the diagnosis (see Figure 10). To avoid the use of `and/or', when it is specified that *either* of two criteria are required, it is always assumed that the presence of *both* criteria also satisfies the requirement.

Detailed criteria for the `unspecified' (.9) categories of the overall ICD-10 chapter V(F) classification are not provided. For the .8 category there are often specific criteria provided by research groups interested in the disorder. Since they are rarely generally known or used and since conditions which would be classified as `other' by definition have lesser public health significance, there are usually no criteria under .8 in the DCR.

The DCR does not contain extensive rules on mutual exclusions since different research projects may have different criteria depending on their objectives. However, some of the more obvious and more frequently used exclusion clauses have been included in DCR-10 for the convenience of users (Figure 10).

Definitions of remission, relapse and duration of episodes have been provided in the DCR-10 in only a limited number of instances. When the DCR-10 is used in research on patients who also suffer from neurological disorders, researchers may also wish to use the neurological adaptation (ICD-10 NA) (see pages 56–58) and various speciality-based classifications produced by nongovernmental organizations and/or included in the ICD-10 fascicles (see page 72).

As a general rule, interference with the performance of social roles has not been used as a diagnostic criterion in the ICD-10. This rule has been followed in the DCR-10 as far as possible,

F20.0–F20.3 General criteria for paranoid, hebephrenic, catatonic, and undifferentiated schizophrenia

G1. Either at least one of the syndromes, symptoms and signs listed under (1) below, or at least two of the symptoms and signs listed under (2) should be present for most of the time during an episode of psychotic illness lasting for at least 1 month (or at some time during most of the days).

(1) At least one of the following must be present:

(a) thought echo, thought insertion or withdrawal, or thought broadcasting.

(b) delusions of control, influence, or passivity, clearly referred to body or limb movements of specific thoughts, actions, or sensations; delusional perception.

(c) hallucinatory voices giving a running commentary on the patient's behaviour, or discussing the patient among themselves, or other types of hallucinatory voices coming from some part of the body.

(d) persistent delusions of other kinds that are culturally inappropriate and completely impossible (e.g. being able to control the weather, or being in communication with aliens from another world).

(2) or at least two of the following:

(a) persistent hallucinations in any modality, when occurring every day for at least 1 month, when accompanied by delusions (which may be fleeting or half-formed) without clear affective content, or when accompanied by persistent over-valued ideas;

(b) neologisms, breaks or interpolations in the train of thought, resulting in incoherence or irrelevant speech;

(c) catatonic behaviour, such as excitement, posturing, waxy flexibility, negativism, mutism, and stupor;

(d) 'negative' symptoms, such as marked apathy, paucity of speech, and blunting or incongruity of emotional responses (it must be clear that these are not due to depression or to neuroleptic medication).

G2. Most commonly used exclusion clauses

(1) If the patient also meets criteria for manic episode (F30.-) or depressive episode (F32.-), the criteria listed under G1(1) and G1(2) above must have been met before the disturbance of mood developed.

(2) The disorder is not attributable to organic brain disease (in the sense of F00–F09), or to alcohol- or drug-related intoxication (F1x.0), dependence (F1x.2), or withdrawal (F1x.3 and F2x.4).

Continued

F20.0 Paranoid schizophrenia

A. The general criteria for schizophrenia (F20.0–F20.3) must be met.

B. Delusions or hallucinations must be prominent (such as delusions of persecution, reference, exalted birth, special mission, bodily change, or jealousy; threatening or commanding voices, hallucinations of smell or taste, sexual or other bodily sensations).

C. Flattening or incongruity of affect, catatonic symptoms, or incoherent speech must not dominate the clinical picture, although they may be present to a mild degree.

Figure 10. Sample page from DCR version. Reproduced with permission, WHO [14].

but there are a few unavoidable exceptions, the most obvious being simple schizophrenia and dissocial personality disorder. Once the decision had been made to include these disorders in the classification, it was considered best to do so without modifying the concepts; as a consequence it became necessary to include interference with social role in the diagnostic criteria for these disorders. Experience and further research should show whether these decisions were justified.

The field trials carried out to test how reliably psychiatrists can use the classification showed that the reliability of assessment using the DCR was higher than the reliability offered when the CDDG are used (Figure 11). The usefulness and ease of employing the criteria were also examined by psychiatrists in a number of countries. The results in Figure 12 indicate that there were rarely any problems with the use of diagnostic criteria.

The DCR have been incorporated in the algorithms accompanying the assessment instruments and their application can ensure that the groups of patients selected for a particular research project will be homogenous in so far as their symptoms and clinical pictures are concerned.

The use of criteria and rules indicated in the DCR is a convention which should enable investigators to compose groups

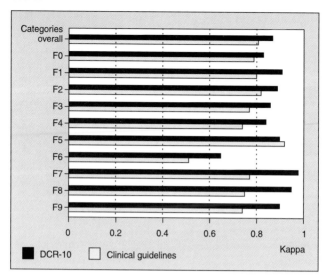

Figure 11. Interrater reliability (in kappa) of CDDG, compared to DCR.

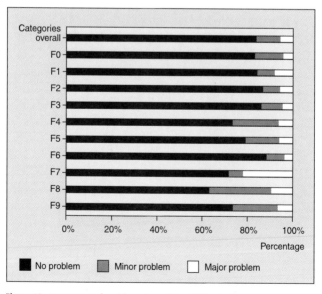

Figure 12. Assessment of problems in applying DCR criteria.

of patients which are symptomatologically similar. It is, however, important to underline that in the majority of instances there is no solid evidence about the equiponderation of criteria, nor about the numbers of symptoms that belong to the `true' diagnosis of the condition. Similarly, in most instances the duration of symptoms required for a positive rating on any one criterion is defined in accordance with practical experience and this may be subject to more variations than the duration of incubation for an infectious disease, for example.

There is no harm and much to gain from the use of standard criteria and conventions as long as it is remembered that these are *conventions* which are not immutable and which may well have to change in the light of results of scientific investigations and accumulation of new observations. The fact that a condition is precisely described does not make it a disease satisfying all the requirements for the definition of a disease — which should have a well-established aetiology and pathogenesis, well-described symptoms, predictable reactions to treatment, a foreseeable course and a probable outcome — it just helps to promote understanding among those who are concerned with research, education and care for people suffering from mental disorders.

Chapter 5

MULTIAXIAL VERSION OF THE ICD-10 CLASSIFICATION OF MENTAL DISORDERS

For certain purposes and in certain situations it is advantageous to employ a multiaxial classification, that is, a classification which allows simultaneous assessment of different aspects of the patient's illness. Planning for care has to take into account not only the clinical psychiatric syndrome but also the intellectual level of the patient, the social circumstances in which the patient lives and any other diseases or impairments from which he or she may suffer. In scientific investigations of outcome or duration of illness it is also of importance to obtain information about levels of impairment and disability and change over time, and about the patients' environment so as to be able to interpret the results obtained. In education about psychiatric illness (and illness in general) a key requirement is to ensure that medical (undergraduate and postgraduate) students continuously examine the patients' illness in the context of genetic, social and environmental factors which affect the patient, their illness and the possibilities for its treatment.

The WHO was therefore interested in studies which would allow it to examine whether the application of a multiaxial approach to diagnosis is possible in different service and research situations and in different cultural settings. A first attempt to obtain information about this issue was the exploration of the usefulness and applicability of a multiaxial classification of mental disorders in childhood. During the third meeting of Programme A (see page 13) in Paris in 1967 the advantages of a multiaxial system were debated at length and a recommendation was made which led to tests of the proposals presented in Paris [26] and to the publication of the multiaxial scheme for childhood mental disorders by WHO a few years later [27]. This scheme was subsequently used in other settings and further developed. At present, the childhood mental disorders classification has six axes:

Axis I   Clinical psychiatric syndrome

Axis II   Specific disorders of psychological development

Axis III   Intellectual level

Axis IV   Medical conditions

Axis V   Associated abnormal psychosocial situations

Axis VI   Global assessment of disability.

A publication, in book form, of the multiaxial classification for the assessment of mental disorders in children (together with the results of the field tests) is expected in 1995.

In adult psychiatry the first proposals for a multiaxial ICD-10 version were also made long ago. The discussions about the classification of mental disorders in old age held during the Programme A meeting in Moscow in 1969 produced a number of recommendations about the classification of mental disorders in old age and suggested that a multiaxial classification of mental disorders in old age accompanying the ICD-8 should be produced and tested. The axes were to serve for the recording of the clinical psychiatric syndrome, of the (cognitive) impairment and of the disability linked to mental illness. These proposals were not taken up for a variety of reasons, but several years later another multiaxial classification was proposed for use in primary health care [28].

In the course of the development of the ICD-10, a proposal for a multiaxial presentation of the ICD-10 classification of mental disorders was produced and tested. This proposal for a multiaxial presentation of the ICD-10 has introduced several significant innovations which distinguish it from other multiaxial classification. First, the classification proposes to code all medical conditions — psychiatric disorders as well as any other disease — on the same axis (Axis 1). Modern information processing technology makes the retrieval of several diagnostic statements from the same axis easy, thus eliminating the earlier arguments against coding several diagnoses on the same axis. The idea to place all diagnoses together has a clear ideological advantage in that it demonstrates, to psychiatrists and nonpsychiatrists, that the distinction between mental and physical disorders is a thing of the past, unnecessary and harmful to the development of both psychiatry and medicine in general. The codes used for the diseases to be placed on this axis are the codes from chapters I–XIX (A00–Y98), i.e. the chapters serving to record diseases in the ICD-10.

The second axis of the classification deals with the disability (see page 32 for a discussion on the use of the term `disability') due to impairments produced by the illness (or illnesses) from which the individual suffers. The instruction to the user of the classification is to assess the total disability present without attempting to guess how much of it is due to each of the diseases (if the patient suffers from more than one disorder). The ratings are made on a five-point scale for four areas of functioning (e.g. work).

The third axis serves to record environmental factors and personal life factors which influence the course and outcome of the disease. The choice of items which should be examined on this axis has been determined by epidemiological evidence and clinical practice. The codes on that axis correspond to codes in Chapter XXI(Z) and their description is made in accordance with the content of each of the codes (on the four-character level) in the ICD. The triaxial classification for use in adult psychiatry shown in Figure 13 has been tested in more than 30 countries and the results of the trials in terms of reliability among users, cross-cultural applicability and ease of use will be published in 1995.

Axis I   Clinical diagnosis
             Mental as well as physical disorders catalogued in ICD-10
             are recorded on this axis

Axis II   Disabilities
             Disabilities resulting from mental and/or physical disorders
             are recorded on this axis. They are rated in respect of:
             - Personal care and survival
             - Occupational functioning
             - Functioning with family and household members
             - Broader social behaviour (e.g. leisure activities)

Axis III   Contextual factors (selected Z codes)
             Factors contributing to the presentation or course of the
             disorder(s) are recorded on this axis. The following groups
             of factors are covered by Axis III:
             Problems related to negative life events in childhood
             Problems related to education and literacy
             Problems related to primary support group, including
                 family circumstances
             Problems related to the social environment
             Problems related to housing or economic circumstances
             Problems related to (un)employment
             Problems related to physical environment
             Problems related to legal circumstances
             Problems related to family history of diseases or
                 disabilities
             Problems related to lifestyle

Figure 13. The multiaxial presentation of the ICD-10 for use in the diagnosis of
mental disorders of the adult.

Chapter 6

THE PRIMARY HEALTH CARE (PHC) VERSION OF THE ICD-10 CLASSIFICATION OF MENTAL DISORDERS

The Primary Health Care (PHC) version of the ICD-10 has been produced in recognition of the vast amount of evidence showing that a large majority of people with psychiatric disorders seek help for their disease from general practitioners and other primary health care staff. It was therefore of importance to offer the general health care worker a possibility to record mental and behavioural disorders in a convenient manner, and necessary to do everything possible to facilitate the use of a classification of mental disorders in primary health care. General practitioners are busy people and it is unlikely that they would agree to undergo long additional training in the use of the classification. This means that the classification had to be almost self-explanatory, it had to use terms with which general practitioners are familiar and it had to concentrate on conditions frequently seen in general health care. The time that practitioners are able to devote to a patient is also very limited and it was therefore necessary to ensure that the classification is easy to use. Furthermore, in order to be able to use the reports for public health purposes it was necessary to make the classification for primary care fully compatible with the ICD-10. Finally, it is very likely that general practitioners will be more inclined to use the classification if they can see an immediate and direct benefit from its use. It was therefore decided to produce a guide to the diagnosis and management of the patient to accompany each of the disorders included in the PHC classification.

The first task placed before the group drafting this version of the ICD-10 classification of mental and behavioural disorders was to select categories which will be included in it. After considerable discussion it was agreed to produce a classification containing ICD-10 categories which refer to conditions of major public health importance, about whose definition and treatment there is international consensus and for which there is an acceptable and effective treatment. This helped to reduce the number of categories; in the field trial version of the PHC classification only 24 categories were proposed and it is possible that this number will be further reduced. The field trials were being run in the languages of the countries participating in the trials and involved general practitioners as well as psychiatrists. These trials have been under way for nearly a year and their results seem to support the choice of categories made using the principles listed above. The categories selected for the field trials are shown in Figure 14.

Each of the categories is printed on a card and accompanied by a set of guidelines about the identification (Figure 15) and management (Figure 16) of the condition. Examples of cards used for the category of depression are shown on pages 53–55.

In addition to the flipcards, the ICD-10 classification kit for use in primary health care will also contain *flow charts* leading the practitioner from the symptom to the possible choice of diagnoses, and *educational materials* which the general practitioner may wish to give to their patients to provide them with information about their diseases and their management.

The classification of mental disorders for use in primary health care is different from the other versions of the ICD in that it is expected that there will be considerable additions to or changes of the original materials in the course of preparation of the texts which will be used in different countries. While the list of categories is unlikely to change (except possibly being enlarged or reduced in accordance with national needs) the cards giving suggestions about the recognition of the disorders and their treatment will have to be adjusted to conditions prevailing in the countries and services in which the classification will be used. The first results of trials show, for example, that general practitioners in different countries recommended changes and clarifications to several of the identification and management cards, but they did so for different cards in various countries.

Organic disorders (F0)

Dementia	F00
Delirium	F05

Psychoactive substance abuse (F1)

Alcohol use disorders	F10
Drug use disorders	F11
Tobacco use disorders	F17.1

Psychotic disorders (F2)

Acute psychotic disorders	F23
Chronic psychotic disorders	F20

Mood, stress-related and anxiety disorders (F3 & 4)

Bipolar disorder	F31
Depression	F32
Phobic disorders	F40
Panic disorders	F41.0
Generalized anxiety	F41.1
Mixed anxiety and depression	F41.2
Adjustment disorder	F43
Dissociative (conversion) disorders	F44
Unexplained somatic complaints	F45
Neurasthenia	F48.0

Physiological disorders (F5)

Eating disorders	F50
Sexual disorders	F52
Sleep problems	F51

Mental retardation (F7)

Mental retardation	F70

Childhood and adolescence (F9)

Hyperkinetic disorder	F90
Conduct disorders of childhood	F91
Enuresis	F98

Figure 14. The categories used in the field trials for the Primary Health Care version of the ICD-10 classification of mental disorders.

Presenting complaints

May present initially with one or more physical symptoms (fatigue, pain).
Further enquiry will reveal depression or loss of interest

Sometimes presents as irritability

Diagnostic features

Low or sad mood

Loss of interest or pleasure

Associated symptoms are frequently present:
Disturbed sleep
Guilt or low self-worth
Fatigue or loss of energy
Poor concentration
Disturbed appetite
Suicidal thoughts or acts

Movements and speech may be slowed, but may also appear agitated

Symptoms of anxiety or nervousness are frequently also present

Differential diagnosis

If hallucinations (hearing vocies, seeing visions) or delusions (strange or unusual beliefs) are present, see also card on Acute Psychotic disorders F23* about these problems

If history of manic episode (excitement, elevated mood, rapid speech) is present, see card on Bipolar disorder F31

If heavy alcohol use is present, see card on Alcohol Use Disorders F10, Drug Disorders F10*

Figure 15. Example of a draft diagnostic card for depression (F32*) used in the field trials of the PHC version of the ICD-10 MNH. Reproduced with permission, WHO.

Essential information for patient and family

i. Depression is common and effective treatments are available

ii. Depression is not weakness or laziness; patients are trying their hardest

Specific counselling to patient and family

i. Ask about risk of suicide. Can the patient be sure of not acting on suicidal ideas? Close supervision by family or friends may be needed

ii. Plan short-term activities which give enjoyment or build confidence

iii. Advise patients to resist pessimism and self-criticism; not to act on pessimistic ideas (e.g. ending marriage, leaving job); and not to concentrate on negative or guilty thoughts

iv. If physical symptoms are present, discuss link between physical symptoms and mood (see card on Unexplained Somatic Complaints F45*)

v. After improvement, discuss signs of relapse, plan with patient action to be taken if signs of relapse occur

Medication

i. Consider antidepressant drugs if sad mood or loss of interest are prominent for at least 2 weeks and 4 or more of these symptoms are present:

Fatigue or loss of energy

Guilt or self-reproach

Thoughts of death or suicide

Agitation or slowing of movement and speech

Disturbed speech

Poor concentration

Disturbed appetite

If there was good response to one drug in the past, use that again.

If older or medically ill, use medication with fewer side-effects

If anxious or unable to sleep, use more sedating drug

ii. Build up to effective dose, use lower doses if older or medically ill.

iii. Explain how medication should be used:

Medication should be taken every day

Improvement will build over 2–3 weeks

Mild side-effects will occur and usually fade in 7–10 days

Check with the doctor before stopping medication

iv. Continue antidepressant for at least 3 months after symptoms improve

Continued

Specialist consultation

i. If suicide risk is severe, consider consultation and hospitalization

ii. If significant depression persists, consider consultation about other therapies

iii. More intensive psychotherapies (e.g. cognitive therapy) may be useful for acute treatment and relapse prevention

Figure 16. Example of a draft management card for depression (F32*), as used in the field trials of the PHC version of the ICD-10 MNH. Reproduced with permssion, WHO.

It will therefore be necessary to establish a continuing dialogue between the WHO and the centres which will adapt the classification for national use, to ensure that the changes which they propose do not unduly disrupt the comparability of the results of the classification. The ICD centres which have collaborated with the WHO in the production of the classification will have to play an important role in this process, not only because of their vast experience in matters concerning the classification of mental disorders and their familiarity with local conditions but also because of the necessity to prepare the texts in languages which primary health care workers can easily use. It is also proposed to intensify the process of consultation about the best way to identify and treat mental illness in different settings by suggesting that the classification be discussed at joint meetings of nongovernmental organizations representing general practitioners and psychiatrists. They will have the classification and the materials which accompany it as models for the development of similar products at national level. They will also be invited to assume leadership in the organization of training and information activities facilitating the use of the classification. It is expected that the field tests that are being carried out at present will produce not only results about the value of the classification, its acceptability, goodness of fit and other features but also provide useful suggestions about the best ways to carry out education about the classification and its use at the local level.

Chapter 7

THE PSYCHIATRIC AND NEUROLOGICAL ADAPTATIONS OF THE ICD-10

The Psychiatric Adaptation of the ICD-10 (ICD-10 PA) and the Neurological Adaptation of the ICD-10 (ICD-10 NA) are in preparation and will be published in 1995. The first, the ICD-10 PA, is primarily intended for use by those in charge of coding diagnostic statements in psychiatric services and in other services in which psychiatric disorders are frequently seen. It contains all the codes from Chapter V(F) on mental and behavioural disorders with their brief glossary notes; a listing of other ICD codes likely to be frequently used in mental health care facilities; the conversion tables allowing the translation of codes between the eighth, ninth and 10th revisions of the ICD; and a detailed index of all the diagnostic terms contained in the volume. The ICD-10 PA will also contain the translation of ICD-10 codes into codes of the clinical modification of the ICD-9 (the ICD-9 CM), which is currently still being used in a number of countries, and in later editions the ICD-10 CM (should this be produced). The ICD-10 PA will also include other materials (such as explanations of various conventions governing the use of codes in the ICD) likely to be of use to coders.

The Neurological Adaptation of the ICD-10 (ICD-10 NA) is composed in a different manner and its main purposes are different from those of the ICD-10 PA. It will contain instructions and recommendations for the use of the ICD-10 NA and a list of neurological disorders; sizeable extracts from other parts of the ICD-10 likely to be of use in neurological practice, including the classification of neoplasms by morphology; and an index. What makes it different from the ICD-10 PA is the manner in which the ICD-10 NA has been produced and the manner in which it will be used. The ICD-10 PA list of psychiatric categories is a direct reprint of Chapter V(F) which is also contained in the main body of the ICD-10; the ICD-10 NA listing of categories contains a comprehensive listing of neurological disorders, syndromes and named diseases, ordered by ICD-10 code number. The terms which have been included in the list have been assembled by a core group of experts in collaboration with a variety of nongovernmental professional organizations, in particular the World Federation of Neurology and the classification committee of the American Academy of Neurology (see Figure 17) [29]. The multitude of terms included often required the use of fifth, sixth and seventh characters in the ICD-10 and the listing, which was produced through the process of extensive consultation with experts, specialist institutions and professional organizations, is one of the most comprehensive assemblies of diagnostic terms used in neurology produced so far. It is planned to develop glossary definitions for some groups of disorders such as headaches, and to include them in the body of the ICD-10 after field testing and further consultation. There is as yet no target date for this ambitious undertaking, which will require work similar in nature to that which had to be undertaken to produce the glossary which accompanies categories in Chapter V(F) of the ICD-10.

In terms of probable main users of the ICD-10 NA and the ICD-10 PA there is also a difference; the former will most likely be used by specialists in neurology, neurosurgery and other applied neuroscientific disciplines, while the latter will mainly be used by coders. Specialists in psychiatry will mainly use the CDDG, DCR and multiaxial presentations of the ICD-10 classification of mental disorders.

G43	Migraine
	Use additional external cause code (Ch.XX) if desired to identify drug, if drug-induced
	Excludes: headache NOS (R51); atypical facial pain (G50)
G43.0	Migraine without aura (common migraine)
G43.1	Migraine with aura (classical migraine)
G43.10	With typical aura
G43.11	with prolonged aura
G43.12	With acute onset aura

Use sixth character, if desired, to identify neurological symptoms

G43.1x0	Hemianopic and other visual migraine
G43.1x1	Hemisensory migraine
G43.1x2	Migraine with aphasia
G43.1x3	Basilar migraine
G43.1x4	Migraine aura (all types) without headache
G43.1x5	Familial hemiplegic migraine
G43.1x7	Multiple types of aura
G43.1x8	Other specified migraine with aura

Figure 17. Example of a category in the ICD-10 NA. Reproduced with permission, WHO [4].

Chapter 8

INSTRUMENTS FOR THE ASSESSMENT OF MENTAL STATE AND OF OTHER PATIENT CHARACTERISTICS

The agreement among mental health workers about criteria which have to be fulfilled to make a particular diagnosis is not a guarantee that the same conditions will be called the same name. To be certain that this will happen it is necessary to standardize the collection of data on the basis of which it will be decided whether the requirements specified in the criteria are satisfied. The past several decades witnessed significant progress in the methods which can be used to obtain data that will be comparable despite being collected in different social settings. Several major studies, such as those coordinated by the WHO to explore the form, frequency and outcome of severe mental disorders, demonstrated that instruments for the collection of transculturally comparable data can be produced, that psychiatrists and other mental health workers from different cultures can be trained in their use to make reliable assessments of the mental state and other characteristics of patients, and that data collected in this way can be computer-processed in a way that leads to the assignment of cases to diagnostic categories contained in the ICD.

Among the many instruments which the WHO has produced and tested [30] three have been produced in conjunction with the development of the ICD-10 and serve to collect data which can be used to arrive at an assignment to an ICD-10 (and DSM-III and DSM-IV) categories. These are the *Composite International Diagnostic Interview* (CIDI), *Schedule for Clinical Assessment in Neuropsychiatry* (SCAN), and the *International Personality Disorder Examination* (IPDE).

Composite International Diagnostic Interview (CIDI)

The name of this instrument reflects its origins: the CIDI was developed on the basis of the Diagnostic Interview Schedule through a series of consultations and field studies involving a large number of researchers in many countries [19]. The CIDI was tested in a number of languages and its reliability and applicability in different settings is well documented.

CIDI is an instrument that can be used by interviewers after a relatively brief training. It is a highly structured instrument intended for use by trained lay interviewers and in epidemiological studies of mental disorders in general populations. CIDI questions are fully spelled out and positive answers are further explored with a strictly specified probing system, which allows the interviewer to obtain the information necessary for determining the psychiatric significance of a reported phenomenon. A symptom is considered of psychiatric relevance if a doctor has ever attributed a psychological aetiology to it, found no physical basis for it, or if the respondent reports that there was at least one occasion when its occurrence was not explained by a physical illness or condition, an injury, or use of alcohol, drugs or other medication. The symptom is considered clinically significant if it led to professional consultation, treatment with medication, or was believed by the respondent to have interfered significantly with life or activities.

The instrument consists of 288 symptom questions, but because of skip rules not all of them are asked of every respondent. It further incorporates questions for the assessment of the first and last occurrence of a symptom (onset and recency questions) and items for determination of duration and frequency of selected symptoms and syndromes.

The CIDI package consists of the following components:

- Interview schedule
- Researcher's manual
- Training manual

- Computer manual

- Data entry and computer scoring programmes

- Computerized CIDI (CIDI-Auto).

Proper training is a prerequisite for using CIDI. The researcher's manual, interviewer's manual and other associated training materials are used in providing that training. CIDI computer programmes enable users to enter, clear and score the interview and are available on a floppy disk for use with an IBM-compatible personal computer. The computer manual explains how to use the computer programmes and algorithms.

A number of versions and modules of the CIDI have been developed. A list of some of these versions and modules is given in Figure 18, and a sample page from CIDI is shown in Figure 19.

Version	Description
Computerized CIDI (CIDI-Auto):	CIDI questions appearing on a computer screen. Can be used by interviewers or treating physicians.
Quick CIDI:	A version accompanied by a programme that interrupts the interview as soon as a sufficient amount of information to make a diagnosis has been assembled.
CIDI Primary Health Care Version (CIDI-PHC):	Includes some of the CIDI sections and some new sections.
CIDI Substance Abuse Module (CIDI-SAM):	Can be used on its own or together with the CIDI.

Figure 18. Selected CIDI versions and modules.

			I EVER	II WORST
LOST INTEREST				NO YES

DEPICDB2 DYSICDC6	E19	Has there ever been **a period** of several weeks when your **interest in sex was** [Was your interest in sex] a lot **less than usual**?	PRB: 1 3 4 5*6	1 5
		MD:............ OTHER:............		
		IF NO INTEREST EVER, CODE PRB 6 AND SKIP TO E20. IF NOT CODED PRB 5*, SKIP TO E20.		
DEPICDS8		A. Did you ever [Did you] completely lose your interest in sex?	NO ....1 YES.......5	1 5

DYSICDC6 MEL3R1 DEP3RA2 DEPICDB2	E20	Has there ever been two weeks or longer when you **lost** [Did you lose] **interest in most things** like work or hobbies or things you usually liked to do for fun?	PRB: 1 3 4 5*6	1 5
		MD:............ OTHER:............		
		IF NOT CODED PRB 5*, SKIP TO E21.		
DEPICDS1		A. Did you ever [Did you] completely lose all interest in things like work or hobbies or things you usually liked to do for fun?	NO ....1 YES.......5	1 5

| MEL3R2
DEPICDS2 | E21 | Have you ever had 2 weeks or longer when you lost [Did you lose] the ability to enjoy having good things happen to you, like winning something or being praised or complimented? | | 1   5 |

Figure 19. A sample page from CIDI. Reproduced with permission, WHO [31].

Schedule for Clinical Assessment in Neuropsychiatry (SCAN)

SCAN is a set of instruments aimed at assessing, measuring and classifying the psychopathology and behaviour associated with the major psychiatric disorders of adult life. It consists of:

(i) a structured clinical interview schedule with semi-standardized probes, i.e. the 10th edition of Present State Examination (PSE-10); (ii) glossary with symptom definitions; (iii) Item Group Checklist (IGC); and (iv) Clinical History Schedule (CHS). The instrument is intended for use by clinicians (psychiatrists or clinical psychologists) after training in its application. The administration time is 60–90 minutes.

SCAN was developed in collaboration with experts from many countries, from the original schedule for the assessment of the Present State Examination (PSE) [32]. A sample page is shown overleaf (Figure 20) The PSE-10, which is at the core of the SCAN, has demonstrated its value in the course of numerous studies in different countries. PSE-10 has two main parts. Part 1 includes nonpsychotic sections covering worrying, tension, panic, anxiety and phobias, obsessional symptoms, depressed mood and ideation, impaired thinking, concentration, energy interests, bodily functions, weight, sleep and eating disorders, alcohol and drug abuse. Part 2 contains sections covering psychotic and cognitive disorders and abnormalities of behaviour, speech and affect. Both parts allow rating of other episodes or `lifetime' manifestations in addition to present state ratings.

The Item Group Checklist (IGC) is a list of 59 item groups rated on the basis of information derived from case notes and informants.

The Clinical History Schedule (CHS) consists of sections on childhood and education to age 16, intellectual level, social roles and performance, and social handicap. Information about disorders of adult personality and behaviour, and physical illnesses or disabilities not entered elsewhere can also be recorded here.

The SCAN Glossary is an essential part of SCAN. It provides definitions of symptoms and signs to be assessed by the interviewer. Data from all schedules are coded on a set of scoring sheets. A diagnostic computer programme is available to process the data. A computerized version of the SCAN (CAPSE) is being prepared.

10.003 Duration of expansive or irritable mood

1 Present, but less than four days.
2 Present at least 4 days consecutively.
3 Present, at least 1 week.
4 Present more than 2 months.
5 Hospital admission required irrespective of duration.

If > 2 years, consider cyclothymia [See note at the top of Section].

CUT OFF => to 11.001 if 10.001, 10.002, 10.003, 3.009 and 3.011 all rated 0.

10.004 Pressing and racing thoughts

Do you find thoughts crowding into and racing through your mind - as though they were speeded up and you had too many thoughts compared with usual - during [PERIOD]?

- Could you describe that?
- How long did it last?

Use SCALE I

10.005 Overtalkativeness

Have people said that you talked too fast and too much so that they couldn't understand you? Or do you feel pressure to keep talking?

Use SCALE I

If > 2 years, consider cyclothymia.

10.006 Distractibility

Have you found that you could not keep your attention on one subject long enough to deal with it properly?

– That your attention keeps being distracted by irrelevant things happening around you?

Use SCALE I

If > 2 years, consider cyclothymia.

Figure 20. A sample page from SCAN. Reproduced with permission, WHO.

There are also numerous similarities between the SCAN and the CIDI. These include the form of output (ICD-10 and DSM-IV diagnostic assignment), the form and duration of training (approximately 5 days), the availability of the instruments in many languages and the existence of a network of centres which can help by training new users of the instrument and by providing advice to those who wish to use the instrument in studies. Both instruments are available in many languages. The major differences between CIDI and SCAN are summarized in Figure 21.

CIDI	SCAN
Fully structured	Semi-structured
Non-clinician application	Clinician applications
Probe-flow prescribed	Cross-examination
Ratings based on subject's answers	Ratings based on interviewer's judgement about the presence of symptoms
Choice of items decided on the basis of their necessity for the assessment of whether criteria for diagnosis have been met	Choice of items decided by the aim to obtain a comprehensive psychopathological assessment

Figure 21. The major differences between CIDI and SCAN.

The International Personality Disorder Examination (IPDE)

The International Personality Disorder Examination (IPDE) bears a close resemblance to the Personality Disorder Examination (PDE) from which it was developed in the course of an international study [34]. The IPDE assesses phenomenology and life experiences relevant to the diagnosis of personality disorders according to ICD-10, DSM-III-R and DSM-IV criteria. Each criterion is precisely defined, and guidelines and anchor-points for scoring are provided for each IPDE question. The instrument is intended for use by clinicians (psychiatrists or clinical psychologists) experienced in the assessment of personality disorders.

The latest version of IPDE consists of 153 items which are arranged under the following six headings: work, self, interpersonal relationships, affects, reality testing and impulse control. The items are introduced by open-ended inquiries that offer the individual an opportunity to discuss the topic before answering, and then to supplement the answers with examples or anecdotes. In addition, the interview provides a set of probes to determine whether the individual has met the requirements of frequency, duration and age of onset. IPDE adopts two rating conventions: a symptom is rated positive if it existed for at least five years and a disorder can be rated positive if at least one criterion has been met prior to age 25.

The IPDE covers the following diagnoses of personality disorders: paranoid, schizoid, schizotypal, antisocial, borderline, histrionic, compulsive, passive–aggressive, sadistic, self-defeating, not otherwise specified.

Two versions of the IPDE are currently in use and will be published shortly, one to produce diagnoses according to the ICD-10 and another providing DSM-IV assignments. In addition, there is a working version which allows categorization in terms of both classifications, a screener version for diagnoses in accordance with the III.R. revision of the DSM and a clinical adaptation (in Dutch only).

The IPDE has been field tested and was found to be reliable and applicable in different cultures. A sample page from the IPDE is shown in Figure 22.

 Disability Assessment Schedule (DAS)

The Disability Assessment Schedule (DAS) [35] serves to evaluate social functioning, and some of the factors influencing it, in patients with one or more impairments, usually due to mental disorders. It is a semi-structured interview, to be used by psychiatrists, psychologists, sociologists or social workers, after appropriate training.

The instrument is based on the assumption that impairment and disability can be seen and rated relatively independently from symptoms of illness. It consists of 97 items which are accommodated in five parts:

Part 1: *Overall behaviour*, which includes patient's self-care during past month, under-activity, slowness, social withdrawal.

> Marked and persistent identity distur-
> bance manifested by uncertainty about
> preferred values DSM-III-R Borderline:
> 6 (partial)
>
> 20.   0 1 2 ?   0 1 2 ?
>
> Disturbances in and uncertainty about
> internal preferences ICD-10 Emotionally
> Labile: 6 (partial)

Do you have trouble deciding what's important in life?
If Yes: How does that affect you or the way you live your life?

Do you have trouble deciding what's right and wrong?
If Yes: How does that affect you or the way you live your life?

In this context 'values' refers both to issues of ethics and mortality
('right and wrong') and to what is important in life. For a positive score
both are not required. The subject may qualify for either element of the
criterion in two ways. He may report that he is so uncertain about this
values that it causes subjective distress or problems in social or occupational functioning. Or he may, with or without acknowledgement or
awareness of uncertainty about this values, demonstrate the phenomenon by extremely erratic or inconsistent behaviour indicative of uncertain values.

2. Obvious and well documented persistent uncertainty about values as
described above.

1. Probable but less well documented or persistent uncertainty about
values as described above.

0. Absent, doubtful, or not well supported by examples.

Figure 22. A sample page from IPDE. Reproduced with permission, WHO.

Part 2: *Social role performance* — participation in household
activities, marital role, parental role, heterosexual role, social
contacts, occupational role, interests and information, behaviour in emergencies or crisis situations.

Part 3: *Patient in hospital.* This includes ward behaviour,
slowness of movement, over-activity, conversation, social
withdrawal, leisure interests, irrelevant talk, posturing and
mannerisms, violent behaviour, tendency to remain in bed,

personal appearance, behaviour at meal time, nurses' opinion, patient's occupations, contact with outside world.

Part 4: *Modifying factors,* such as specific assets and specific liabilities, home atmosphere, outside support.

Part 5: *Global evaluation of disability.*

Part 6: *Summary.*

The information to rate the patient's functioning is collected from a key informant, from the patient or from written records. Each item in sections 1 and 2 has to be rated on a six-point scale from no dysfunction to maximum dysfunction. For most of the items, patient's current functioning during the previous month should be evaluated against the presumed `average' or `normal' functioning of a person of the same sex, comparable age and social background. A sample page from DAS is shown in Figure 23.

ICD-10 Symptom Checklist

The ICD-10 Symptom Checklist [21] is a semi-structured instrument which clinicians can use in the course of their examination of patients, in order to arrive at a diagnosis which can be in the F0–F6 categories of the ICD-10 Classification of Mental and Behavioural Disorders. It is essentially a listing, by F categories, of the symptoms which should be considered in deciding whether ICD-10 criteria have been met. It requires the clinician to phrase the necessary symptom questions and to probe positive responses to confirm clinical relevance and severity. This is the type of examination clinicians routinely conduct; the difference is that the examination is guided, so that the oversight and other reasons for the unreliability of an unstructured interview are less likely to occur.The symptoms in the Checklist are grouped into: (i) symptoms characterizing organic mental and psychoactive substance use syndromes (F0/F1 module); (ii) symptoms defining psychotic and affective syndromes (F2/F3 module); (iii) symptoms of neurotic and behavioural

2. Social role performance

2.1 Participation in household activities during past month

Card 1
Column

Inquire about:

(i) patient's participation in common activities of the household, such as having meals together, doing domestic chores, going out or visiting together, playing games, watching television, etc.;

(ii) patient's participation in decision-making concerning the household, e.g., decisions about the children, money, etc. For housewives, consider the household jobs that a housewife usually has to do. Make a rating without regard to whether patient is asked to participate, left on his/her own or rejected in some way.

38

Rate 8 if information not available and 9 if item not applicable

No dysfunction: patient participates in household activities about as much as is expected for his/her age, sex, position in the household, and sociocultural context.   0

Minimum dysfunction: patient participates less than would be expected and has little interest in (ii), although such participation would normally be expected for someone in similar circumstances.   1

Obvious dysfunction: household participation is reduced to a narrow range of family functions, performed somewhat incompetently.   2

Serious dysfunction: lack of participation and of competence in household matters, to the extent of being excluded from decision-making by other members.   3

Very serious dysfunction: takes no part in any common activities; is alienated from daily routine; exists alongside the household as a unit.   4

Maximum dysfunction: patient totally excludes himself/herself, or is excluded, from participation in any common household activities; disrupts the functioning of the household as a unit.   5

Figure 23. A sample page from DAS. Reproduced with permission, WHO [35].

syndromes (F4/F5 module); and (iv) symptoms of personality disorders (F6 module). Only those modules for which the patient is screened positive will be used. The interviewer can choose which module will be used.

The checklist lists symptoms and states which, according to the ICD-10 criteria, should be excluded or could be associated with the syndrome. These lists are accompanied by instructions which may help the user in considering other possible syndromes (i.e. differential diagnoses). The checklist also offers the possibility of recording onset, severity and duration of the syndrome as well as the number of episodes. The checklist is accompanied by a glossary, which defines symptoms, signs and other psychopathological terms used in the checklist. The symptom checklist glossary is slightly different but fully compatible with the definitions in the Lexica. An example of a glossary description of an ICD-10 symptom is given in Figure 24, and a sample page is shown in Figure 25.

> Delusion: A false unshakeable belief or judgement, out of keeping with reality and not shared by others with similar sociocultural background to the individual. It is held wth conviction despite evidence which contradicts it. The morbid belief may be about being followed or observed, victimized, persecuted, spouse being unfaithful or may be about self-importance and superiority or about one's own identity or appearance. The theme of the conviction may vary.

Figure 24. Example of ICD-10 Symptom Checklist Glossary definition. Reproduced with permission, WHO.

Symptom checklist

F0/F1 module:
Organic mental and psychoactive substance use syndromes

Organic mental disorders

A. Which of the following symptoms are present?

1. decline in memory ☐
2. decline in other intellectual abilities ☐
3. deterioration in emotional control, social behaviour or motivation ☐
4. impairment of consciousness and attention ☐
5. disturbances of perception or disorientation ☐
6. psychomotor disturbances ☐
7. disturbance of the sleep–wake cycle ☐
8. rapid onset and diurnal fluctuations of symptoms ☐

B. How severe is the syndrome?

— mild ☐
— moderate ☐
— severe ☐

C. What is the onset of the syndrome?

— acute ☐
— chronic ☐

D. What is the duration of the syndrome?

— in days ☐☐
— in months ☐☐
— in years ☐☐

Figure 25. Sample page from the Symptom Checklist. Reproduced with permission, WHO.

Chapter 9

OTHER MEMBERS OF THE ICD-10 MNH FAMILY AND TRAINING MATERIALS

 Fascicles developed for different groups of users

Groups of health workers, members of a subdiscipline and groups of scientists sometimes require a collection of texts specially relevant for their work. Fascicles are intended to deal with such needs. A fascicle is typically a volume containing an abstract of the relevant part of the ICD-10 and materials relevant to the assessment, diagnosis and classification of such a group of disorders. The following fascicles are being developed: cerebrovascular disorders, epilepsy, headaches, hereditary ataxias, movement disorders, multiple sclerosis, pain disorders, mental retardation, psychogeriatrics and sleep disorders. It is expected that the fascicles will have the following components:

i.   An extract from the ICD-10 covering the specific categories of interest

ii.   Diagnostic Criteria for Research for these categories

iii.   List of frequently associated disorders from other parts of the ICD-10

iv.   References to assessment instruments, available in this area

v.   Crosswalks with important national or international classifications in this field

vi.   Other useful information (e.g. list of key publications)

vii.   Index.

In most instances the fascicles will be produced by a non-governmental organization which will also undertake to obtain consensus with other interested groups. Where this is not the case the materials will be written or put together by a group of experts invited to do so by the WHO and then circulated for advice to experts in organizations concerned with mental health.

The International Classification of Impairments, Disabilities and Handicaps

The International Classification of Impairments, Disabilities and Handicaps (ICIDH) has a much shorter history than the ICD. Developed some 15 years ago, it introduced the concept of disablement described on page 32 and proposed a classification which followed this conceptual division [5]. Now that considerable experience has been obtained from the use of the ICIDH it has been decided to produce its second revision, relying on a network of WHO collaborating centres and on collaboration with various nongovernmental organizations.

Lexicons

Definitions of terms used to describe psychiatric syndromes are of as much, if not greater, importance than the description of the syndromes themselves. Aware of this, the WHO has produced three lexicons which accompany the ICD-10 series but can also stand on their own. The first of these, the Lexicon of Psychiatric and Mental Health Terms, was published in 1989 and contains definitions of over 300 terms which appear in Chapter V of the ICD-9 [15]. When the ICD-10 was produced this text was updated and published as its second edition [16]. This not only contains improved formulations for terms in the first edition but also complements these by definitions of other terms used in describing conditions contained in Chapter V(F) and its glossary (Figure 26).

A Lexicon of Alcohol and Drug terms [17] followed. In this instance, the terms included in the ICD-10 short glossary as well as those of importance in the clinical descriptions and diagnostic guidelines were included in the lexicon. The Lexicon of Alcohol and Drug terms did not aim to provide a

> **derealization** A subjective experience of alienation, similar to **depersonalization** but involving the external world rather than the individual's self-experience and personal identity. The surroundings may seem to lack colour and life and appear as artificial or as a stage on which people are acting contrived roles.
> ***See also:*** depersonalization–derealization syndrome

Figure 26. Definition from the Lexicon of Psychiatric and Mental Health Terms. Reproduced with permission, WHO [16].

comprehensive coverage of every term relating to alcohol and drug use. Terms relating to production and marketing, names of specific drugs, slang terms and terms derived or mainly used in particular scientific disciplines were by and large excluded. Historical origins of the terms are usually not given but there are frequently comments on whether the term is favoured, deprecated or obsolete. A lexicon of culture-specific terms has also been drafted and will be published in 1995. In addition to these three lexicons several other lexical documents belong to the ICD-10 mental health family of documents. These include the terms used in the glossary included in the SCAN instruction manual [33] and a dictionary of terms concerning epilepsy [36]. A multilingual dictionary giving translations of the terms in the ICD-10 is also in production (see page 32).

 The ICD-10 Mental Disorder Casebook

The ICD-10 Mental Disorder Casebook contains a number of case histories, of which many were used in the clinical field trials of chapter V(F) of the ICD-10, and in the ICD-10 training courses in the application of the CDDG and DCR. The case histories have been selected with a view to provide examples of clinical conditions and disorders that fit the diagnostic categories of the ICD-10, and between them provide illustrative material for most of the diagnoses that would be classified in chapter V(F). They are presented in the order of the diagnostic classification to make it easier for the reader to identify diagnostic examples, and have been collected from various countries, thus representing different cultures and emphasizing the international nature and the applicability of chapter V(F) of the ICD-10 in different cultures. Each case history contains a short paragraph describing the clinical features of the patient on presentation and a discussion of the diagnosis according to the ICD-10. The book is meant for self-instruction and for use in ICD-10 training courses but may also be of value for medical students, psychiatric social workers, clinical psychologists, psychiatric nurses and nurses' assistants in their training on psychiatry.

Pocket Guide to the ICD-10 Classification of Mental and Behavioural Disorders

This book [25] contains a combination of materials from the short glossary, CDDG and DCR accompanied by notes for users. It also contains a conversion table between Chapter V of the ICD-9 and ICD-10, notes on some of the same problems that are still unresolved, as well as diagnostic notes and comments on points of special interest and importance. Some of these notes are unique to the volume while others have been taken from the CDDG and the DCR.

Training materials

A variety of materials have been prepared for use in ICD-10 training and familiarization courses. These include a collection of scientific papers, summaries of information about specific aspects of the ICD-10, videotaped and written interviews, sample case histories, a list of references to publications concerning the ICD-10, a set of transparencies and slides for use in teaching about the classification and a description of computer programmes related to the ICD. Many of these materials have been translated or produced in languages other than English. The WHO ICD-10 MNH

Training and Reference centres and the World Psychiatric Association play a key role in the production and distribution of these materials.

 'Crosswalks'

In view of the importance of being able to `translate' statistics from one classification period to the other, it was felt that it would be useful to present conversion tables (`crosswalks'), which would allow the translation of data obtained using the ICD-8, -9 or -10 into one another. These conversion tables will be helpful for coders and clinicians in the transition period between the use of the previous and new systems. Crosswalks are also of major importance for longitudinal studies in psychiatry, for the comparison of results of studies carried out using previous revisions with those using the current revision and for the functioning of the psychiatric services. Crosswalks are also being produced between the ICD-10 and national or subspeciality classifications.

A sample page from the crosswalks is shown in Figure 27.

ICD-9		ICD-10	
307	Special symptoms or syndromes not elsewhere classified		
307.0	Stammering and stuttering *Cluttering*	F98.5 F98.6	Stuttering Cluttering
307.1	Anorexia nervosa	F50.0 F50.1	Anorexia nervosa Atypical anorexia nervosa
307.2	Tics	F95.-	Tic disorders
307.3	Stereotyped repetitive movements	F98.4	Stereotyped movement disorders
307.4	Specific disorders of sleep	F51.-	Nonorganic sleep disorders
307.5	Other and unspecified disorders of eating	F50.1 F50.2 F50.3 F50.4	Atypical anorexia nervosa Bulimia nervosa Atypical bulimia nervosa Over-eating associated with other pscyhological disturbances
		F50.5	Vomiting associated with other psychological disturbances
		F50.8 F50.9 F98.2	Other eating disorders Eating disorder, unspecified Feeding disorder of infancy
	Infantile feeding disturbances Pica (in children)	F98.3	Pica of infancy and childhood
307.6	Enuresis	F98.0	Nonorganic enuresis
307.7	Encoresis	F98.1	Nonorganic encopresis
307.8	Psychalgia	F45.4	Persistent somatoform pain disorder
	Tension headache	G44.2	Tension headache
307/9	Other and unspecified	F98.8	Other specified behavioural and emotional disorders with onset occurring in childhood and adolescence
		F98.9	Unspecified behavioural and emotional disorders with onset usually occurring in childhood and adolescence

Figure 27. Example of a page from the crosswalks. Reproduced with permission, WHO.

Chapter 10

PROBLEMS AND ISSUES FOR FUTURE WORK ON THE INTERNATIONAL CLASSIFICATION OF MENTAL DISORDERS

Although the production of the ICD-10 MNH was a major achievement, there are many tasks that the scientific community, practitioners and teachers of psychiatry and governments must undertake to reap the benefits of ICD-10.

- There is much work to do to introduce instruction about the ICD-10 and its use in the training of doctors and of other health personnel concerned with patient care and evaluation.

- It is necessary to ensure that the system for the collection of data recorded in terms of the ICD-10 has a recipient who will ensure that the data which has been accumulated get used in decision-making about health matters, in research into mental illness and in the provision of care to those who suffer from it.

- Ways must be found to maintain the networks of centres, which can assemble comments and experience gained in use of the classification and combine these with results of scientific investigations to update and improve the ICD-10.

- It is necessary to ensure the continuing engagement of the scientific community in improving the classification and instruments which make its use easier and better.

- Continued involvement of major non-governmental organizations (such as the World Psychiatric Association) is needed in the development of new models of classification and in the training of health professionals about their use.

- There is a need to resolve or at least face some fundamental questions about psychiatric classification and the strategy of its further development.

Over the past 20 years major effort has been put into the definition of ever smaller units and categories of mental disorders, using mainly descriptive psychopathological approaches. A great deal has been achieved in this way and there is probably little to be gained by further refinements of the categories and continuous revisions of the classification. Rather, it might be useful to avoid any new major revisions for some time and explore the value of new strategies of classification, based, for example, on results of long-term follow-up studies of mental disorders on reactions to specific types of treatment or on a particular hypothesis about mental functioning.

While these new strategies are being evaluated it will also be necessary to face epistemological questions which arise with regard to current classificatory systems. These include the definition of methods which can be used in assigning weights to diagnostic criteria; the possibility of combining dimensional and categorical approaches to classification; the correspondence of classifications based on clinical criteria and classifications based on physiological criteria; and numerous others.

Mental health services personnel are not the only people who deal with mental disorders. They do, however, have the duty to produce proposals for a common language, including a classification of mental disorders which will be comprehensible and acceptable to others who have to participate in care for the mentally ill and in decisions about the response of societies to mental illness and the problems it produces. A beginning has been made by the production of a classification for use in primary health care and by the current effort to produce a classification of impairments, disabilities and handicaps which will serve as a tool of communication among those concerned with the consequences of mental illness (including those who finance rehabilitative efforts, such as insurance companies). Other bridges will have to be built to ensure collaboration with other scientific disciplines such as anthropology and sociology, professions participating in the provision of mental health services such as social workers and nurses, and professionals working in narrowly defined areas such as sleep disorders. The aforementioned network of centres may play an important role in this respect, because it can coordinate the many agencies and individuals necessary for progress to be made.

REFERENCE LIST

1. World Health Organization: *International Statistical Classification of Diseases and Related Health Problems, Tenth Revision. Three Volumes.* Geneva: WHO; 1992, 1993, 1994.

2. World Health Organization: *Mental disorders: Glossary and guide to their classification in accordance with the Ninth Revision of the International Classification of Diseases.* Geneva: WHO; 1978.

3. World Health Organization: *Application of the International Classification of Diseases to Neurology (ICD-NA).* Geneva: WHO; 1987.

4. World Health Organization: *Application of the International Classification of Diseases to Neurology (ICD-NA). Second Edition.* Geneva: WHO; in press.

5. World Health Organization: *International Classification of Impairments, Disabilities and Handicaps.* Geneva: WHO; 1980.

6. Stengel E: **Classification of mental disorders.** *Bulletin of the WHO* 1960, **21**:601–663.

7. Lin T-Y: **The epidemiological study of mental disorders.** *WHO Chronicle* 1967, **21**:509–516.

8. Sartorius N: **Classification: An international perspective.** *Psychiatric Annals* 1976, **6**:22–35.

9. Sartorius N: **WHO's work on the epidemiology of mental disorders.** *Soc Psychiatry Psychiatr Epidemiol* 1993, **28**:147–155.

10. World Health Organization and Alcohol, Drug Abuse and Mental Health Administration International Congress Series 669: *Mental Disorders: Alcohol- and Drug-Related Problems.* Amsterdam: Excerpta Medica; 1985.

11. Jablensky A, Sartorius N, Hirshfeld R, *et al.*: **Diagnosis and classification of mental disorders and alcohol- and drug-related problems: A research agenda for the 1980's.** *Psychol Med* 1983, **13**:907–921.

12. Sartorius N, Kaelber C, Cooper J, *et al.*: **Progress towards achieving a common language in psychiatry. Results from the ICD-10 clinical field trial of mental and behavioural disorders.** *Arch Gen Psychiatry* 1993, **50**:115–124.

13. World Health Organization: *The ICD-10 Classification of Mental and Behavioural Disorders — Clinical Descriptions and Diagnostic Guidelines.* Geneva: WHO; 1992.

14. World Health Organization: *The ICD-10 Classification of Mental and Behavioural Disorders — Diagnostic Criteria for Research.* Geneva: WHO; 1993.

15. World Health Organization: *Lexicon of Psychiatric and Mental Health Terms, Volume 1.* Geneva: WHO; 1985.

16. World Health Organization: *Lexicon of Psychiatric and Mental Health Terms, 2nd Edition.* Geneva: WHO; 1994.

17. World Health Organization: *Lexicon of Alcohol and Drug Terms.* Geneva: WHO; 1994.

18. Wing JE, Babor T, Brugha T, *et al.*: **SCAN: Schedule for Clinical Assessment in Neuropsychiatry.** *Arch Gen Psychiatry* 1990, **47**:589–593.

19. Robins LN, Wing JE, Wittchen H-U, *et al.*: **The Composite International Diagnostic Interview: An epidemiological instrument suitable for use in**

conjunction with different diagnostic systems and in different cultures. *Arch Gen Psychiatry* 1988, **45**:1069–1077.

20. Loranger AW, Sartorius N, Andreoli A, *et al.*: **The International Personality Disorder Examination (IPDE): The WHO/ADAMHA international pilot study of personality disorders.** *Arch Gen Psychiatry* 1994, **5**:215–224.

21. Janca A, Üstün TB, Early TS, *et al.*: **The ICD Symptom Checklist: A companion to the ICD-10 Classification of Mental and Behavioural Disorders.** *Soc Psychiatry Psychiatr Epidemiol* 1993, **28**:239–242.

22. World Health Organization: *Schizophrenia. An International Follow-up Study.* Chichester: John Wiley & Sons; 1979.

23. Jablensky A, Sartorius N, Ernberg G, *et al.*: **Schizophrenia: Manifestations, Incidence and Course in Different Cultures: A World Health Organization Ten-Country Study.** *Psychological Medicine Monograph Supplement* 20; 1992.

24. Cooper JE: **On the publication of the Diagnostic and Statistical Manual of mental disorders: Fourth edition (DSM-IV).** *Br J Psychiatry* 1995, **166**:4–8.

25. Cooper JE (ed.) *Pocket Guide to the ICD-10 Classification of Mental and Behavioural Disorders, with Glossary and Diagnostic Criteria for Research, ICD-10:DCR-10.* Edinburgh: Churchill Livingstone; 1994.

26. Rutter M, Lebovici S, Eisenberg L: **A tri-axial classification of mental disorders in childhood.** *J Child Psychol Psychiatr* 1969, **10**:41–61.

27. Rutter M, Shatter D, Shepherd M: *A Multi-Axial Classification of Child Psychiatric Disorders.* Geneva: WHO; 1975.

28. Clare A, Gulbinat A, Sartorius N. **A triaxial classification of health problems presenting in primary health care: a World Health Organization Multi-Centre Study.** *Soc Psychiatry Psychiatr Epidemiol* 1992, **27**:108–116.

29. Orgogozo J-M: **La Classification Internationale des Malaides de l'OMS (CIM-10) et son Application à la Neurologie (CIM-10 AN).** *Rev Neurol* 1994, **150**:813–822.

30. Sartorius N, Janca A: **Psychiatric Instruments Developed by the World Health Organization.** *Soc Psychiatry Psychiatr Epidemiol* 1995 (in press).

31. World Health Organization: *Composite International Diagnostic Interview (CIDI) Version 1.1, Interviewer Manual.* Wasington DC: American Psychiatry Press, Inc.:1993;28.

32. Wing JK, Cooper JE, Sartorius N: *Present State Examination.* Cambridge: Cambridge University Press; 1974.

33. World Health Organization: *Schedules for Clinical Assessment in Neuropsychiatry (SCAN) Version 2.0. Manual.* Washington DC: American Psychiatric Press, Inc.; 1994.

34. Loranger AW, Hirshfeld R, Sartorius N, *et al.*: **The WHO/ADAMHA international pilot study of personality disorders: Background and purpose.** *J Pers Disord* 1991, 5 :296–306.

35. World Health Organization: *WHO Psychiatric Disability Assessment Schedule (WHO/DAS).* Geneva: WHO; 1988.

36. Gastaut H, in collaboration with an international group of experts: *Dictionary of Epilepsy. Part I: Definitions.* Geneva: World Health Organization; 1973.

Appendix A

CHAPTER V: MENTAL AND BEHAVIOURAL DISORDERS

When trying to understand the overall structure of the classification, or how disorders are related to each other, it is helpful to be able to see the whole classification at a glance, and also to see it arranged in different degrees of detail. This appendix shows the whole classification, going down to the fifth character whenever it occurs.

 List of categories

(Categories present only in the DCR-10 are marked with a star*)

F00–F09
Organic, including symptomatic, mental disorders

F00   **Dementia in Alzheimer's disease**
F00.0   Dementia in Alzheimer's disease with early onset
F00.1   Dementia in Alzheimer's disease with late onset
F00.2   Dementia in Alzheimer's disease, atypical or mixed type
F00.8   Dementia in Alzheimer's disease, unspecified

F01   **Vascular dementia**
F01.0   Vascular dementia of acute onset
F01.1   Multi-infarct dementia
F01.2   Subcortical vascular dementia
F01.3   Mixed cortical and subcortical vascular dementia
F01.8   Other vascular dementia
F01.9   Vascular dementia, unspecified

F02   **Dementia in other diseases classified elsewhere**
F02.0   Dementia in Pick's disease ˙
F02.1   Dementia in Creutzfeld–Jakob disease
F02.2   Dementia in Huntington's disease
F02.3   Dementia in Parkinson's disease
F02.4   Dementia in human immunodeficiency virus (HIV) disease
F02.8   Dementia in other specified diseases classified elsewhere

F03   **Unspecified dementia**
A fifth character may be used to specify dementia in F00–F03, as follows:

    .x0   Without additional symptoms
    .x1   With other symptoms, predominantly delusional
    .x2   With other symptoms, predominantly hallucinatory
    x3   With other symptoms, predominantly depressive
    x4   With other mixed symptoms

*A sixth character may be used to indicate the severity of the dementia:
    *.xx0 Mild
    *.xx1 Moderate
    *.xx2 Severe

F04   **Organic amnesic syndrome, not induced by alcohol and other psychoactive substances**

F05   **Delirium not induced by alcohol and other psychoactive substances**
F05.0   Delirium, not superimposed on dementia, so described
F05.1   Delirium, superimposed on dementia, so described
F05.8   Other delirium
F05.9   Delirium, unspecified

F06   **Other mental disorders due to brain damage and dysfunction and to physical disease**
F06.0   Organic hallucinosis
F06.1   Organic catatonic disorder

F06.2 Organic delusional (schizophrenia-like) disorder

F06.3 Organic mood (affective) disorder
.30 Organic manic disorder
.31 Organic bipolar disorder
.32 Organic depressive disorder
.33 Organic mixed affective disorder

F06.4 Organic anxiety disorder

F06.5 Organic dissociative disorder

F06.6 Organic emotionally labile (asthenic) disorder

F06.7 Mild cognitive disorder
.70 Not associated with a physical disorder
.71 Associated with a physical disorder

F06.8 Other specified mental disorders due to brain damage and dysfunction and to physical disease

F06.9 Unspecified mental disorders due to brain damage and dysfunction and to physical disease

F07 Personality and behavioural disorders due to brain disease, damage and dysfunction

F07.0 Organic personality disorder

F07.1 Postencephalitic syndrome

F07.2 Postconcussional syndrome

F07.8 Other organic personality and behavioural disorders due to brain disease, damage and dysfunction

F07.9 Unspecified mental disorders due to brain disease, damage and dysfunction

F09 Unspecified organic or symptomatic mental disorder

F10–F19
Mental and behavioural disorders due to psychoactive substance use

F10.- Mental and behavioural disorders due to use of alcohol

F11.- Mental and behavioural disorders due to use of opioids

F12.- Mental and behavioural disorders due to use of cannabinoids

F13.- Mental and behavioural disorders due to use of sedatives or hypnotics

F14.- Mental and behavioural disorders due to use of cocaine

F15.- Mental and behavioural disorders due to use of other stimulants, including caffeine

F16.- Mental and behavioural disorders due to use of hallucinogens

F17.- **Mental and behavioural disorders due to use of tobacco**

F18.- **Mental and behavioural disorders due to use of volatile solvents**

F19.- **Mental and behavioural disorders due to multiple drug use and use of other psychoactive substances**

Four-, five- and six-character categories are used to specify the clinical conditions as follows, and diagnostic criteria particular to each psychoactive substance are provided where appropriate for acute intoxication and withdrawal state:

F1x.0 Acute intoxication
.00 Uncomplicated
.01 With trauma or other bodily injury
.02 With other medical complications
.03 With delirium
.04 With perceptual distortions
.05 With coma
.06 With convulsions
.07 Pathological intoxication

F1x.1 Harmful use

F1x.2 Dependence syndrome
.20 Currently abstinent
.200 Early remission
.201 Partial remission
.202 Full remission
.21 Currently abstinent, but in a protected environment
.22 Currently on a clinically supervised maintenance or replacement regime (controlled dependence)
.23 Currently abstinent, but receiving treatment with aversive or blocking drugs
.24 Currently using the substance (active dependence)
.240 Without physical features
.241 With physical features
.25 Continuous use
.26 Episodic use (dipsomania)

F1x.3 Withdrawal state
.30 Uncomplicated
.31 With convulsions

F1x.4 Withdrawal state with delirium
.41 Without convulsions
.42 With convulsions

F1x.5 Psychotic disorder
.50 Schizophrenia- like
.51 Predominantly delusional
.52 Predominantly hallucinatory
.53 Predominantly polymorphic

.54 Predominantly depressive psychotic

.55 Predominantly manic psychotic symptoms

.56 Mixed

F1x.6 Amnesic syndrome

F1x.7 Psychotic disorder

.70 Flashbacks

.71 Personality or behavioural disorder

.72 Residual affective disorder

.73 Dementia

.74 Other persisting cognitive disorder

.75 Late-onset psychotic disorder

F1x.8 Other mental and behavioural disorders

F1x.9 Unspecified mental and behavioural disorder

F20–F29
Schizophrenia, schizotypal and delusional disorders

F20   Schizophrenia

F20.0   Paranoid schizophrenia

F20.1   Hebephrenic schizophrenia

F20.2   Catatonic schizophrenia

F20.3   Undifferentiated schizophrenia

F20.4   Post-schizophrenic depression

F20.5   Residual schizophrenia

F20.6   Simple schizophrenia

F20.8   Other schizophrenia

F20.9   Schizophrenia, unspecified

A fifth character may be used to classify course:

.x0   Continuous

.x1   Episodic with progressive deficit

.x2   Episodic with stable deficit

.x3   Episodic remittent

.x4   Incomplete remission

.x5   Complete remission

.x8   Other

.x9   Course uncertain, period of observation too short

F21   Schizotypal disorder

F22   Persistent delusional disorders

F22.0   Delusional disorders

F22.8   Other persistent delusional disorders

F22.9   Persistent delusional disorder, unspecified

F23   Acute and transient psychotic disorders

F23.0   Acute polymorphic psychotic disorder without symptoms of schizophrenia

F23.1   Acute polymorphic psychotic disorder with symptoms of schizophrenia

F23.2   Acute schizophrenia-like psychotic disorder

F23.3   other acute predominantly delusional psychotic disorder

F23.8   Other acute and transient psychotic disorder

F23.9   Acute and transient psychotic disorder, unspecified

A fifth character may be used to classify course:

.x0   Without associated acute stress

.x1   With associated acute stress

F24   Induced delusional disorder

F25   Schizoaffective disorders

F25.0   Schizoaffective disorder, manic type

F25.1   Schizoaffective disorder, depressive type

F25.2   Schizoaffective disorder, mixed type

F25.8   Other schizoaffective disorders

F25.9   Schizoaffective disorder, unspecified

*A fifth character may be use to classify the following subtypes:

*.x0   Concurrent affective and schizophrenic symptoms only

*.x.1   Concurrent affective and schizophrenic symptoms plus persistence of the schizophrenic symptoms beyond the duration of the affective symptoms

F28   Other non-organic psychotic disorders

F29   Unspecified non-organic psychosis

F30–F39
Mood (affective) disorders

F30   Manic episode

F30.0   Hypomania

F30.1   Mania without psychotic symptoms

F30.2   Mania with psychotic symptoms

*.20   With mood-congruent psychotic symptoms

*.21   With mood-incongruent psychotic symptoms

F30.8   Other manic episodes

F30.9   Manic episode, unspecified

F31   Bipolar affective disorder

F31.0   Bipolar affective disorder, current episode hypomanic

F31.1	Bipolar affective disorder, current episode manic without psychotic symptoms
F31.2	Bipolar affective disorder, current episode manic with psychotic symptoms
	*.20 With mood congruent psychotic symptoms
	*.21 With mood incongruent psychotic symptoms
F31.3	Bipolar affective disorder, current episode mild or moderate depression
	.30 Without somatic syndrome
	.31 With somatic syndrome
F31.4	Bipolar affective disorder, current episode severe depression without psychotic symptoms
F31.5	Bipolar affective disorder, current episode severe depression with psychotic symptoms
	*.50 With mood-congruent psychotic symptoms
	*.51 With mood-incongruent psychotic symptoms
F31.6	Bipolar affective disorder, current episode mixed
F31.7	Bipolar affective disorder, currently in remission
F31.8	Other bipolar affective disorders
F31.9	Bipolar affective disorder, unspecified

F32 Depressive episode

F32.0	Mild depressive episode
	.00 Without somatic syndrome
	.01 With somatic syndrome
F32.1	Moderate depressive episode
	.10 Without somatic syndrome
	.11 With somatic syndrome
F32.2	Severe depressive episode without psychotic symptoms
F32.3	Severe depressive episode with psychotic symptoms
	*.30 With mood-congruent psychotic symptoms
	*.31 With mood-incongruent psychotic symptoms
F32.8	Other depressive episodes
F32.9	Depressive episode, unspecified

F33 Recurrent depressive disorder

F33.0	Recurrent depressive disorder, current episode mild
	.00 Without somatic syndrome
	.01 With somatic syndrome
F33.1	Recurrent depressive disorder, current episode moderate
	.10 Without somatic syndrome
	.11 With somatic syndrome

F33.2	Recurrent depressive disorder, current episode severe without psychotic symptoms
F33.3	Recurrent depressive disorder, current episode severe with psychotic symptoms
	*.30 With mood-congruent psychotic symptoms
	*.31 With mood-incongruent psychotic symptoms
F33.4	Recurrent depressive disorder, currently in remission
F33.8	Other recurrent depressive disorders
F33.9	Recurrent depressive disorder, unspecified

F34 Persistent mood (affective) disorders

F34.0	Cyclothymia
F34.1	Dysthymia
F34.8	Other persistent mood (affective) disorders
F34.9	Persistent mood (affective) disorder, unspecified

F38 Other mood (affective) disorders

F38.0	= Other single mood (affective) disorders
	.00 Mixed affective episode
F38.1	Other recurrent mood (affective) disorders
	.10 Recurrent brief depressive disorder
F38.8	Other specified mood (affective) disorders

F39 Unspecified mood (affective) disorder

**F40–F48
Neurotic, stress-related and somatoform disorders**

F40 Phobic anxiety disorders

F40.0	Agoraphobia
	.00 Without panic disorder
	.01 With panic disorder
F40.1	Social phobias
F40.2	Specific (isolated) phobias
F40.8	Other phobic anxiety disorders
F40.9	Phobic anxiety disorder, unspecified

F41 Other anxiety disorders

F41.0	Panic disorder (episodic paroxysmal anxiety)
	*.00 Moderate
	*.01 Severe
F41.1	Generalized anxiety disorder

F41.2	Mixed anxiety and depressive disorder
F41.3	Other mixed anxiety disorders
F41.8	Other specified anxiety disorders
F41.9	Anxiety disorder, unspecified

F42   Obsessive–compulsive disorder

F42.0	Predominantly obsessional thoughts or ruminations
F42.1	Predominantly compulsive acts (obsessional rituals)
F42.8	Other obsessive–compulsive disorders
F42.9	Obsessive–compulsive disorder, unspecified

F43   Reaction to severe stress, and adjustment disorders

F43.0	Acute stress reaction
	*.00 Mild
	*.01 Moderate
	*.02 Severe
F43.1	Post-traumatic stress disorder
F43.2	Adjustment disorders
	.20 Brief depressive reaction
	.21 Prolonged depressive reaction
	.22 Mixed anxiety and depressive reaction
	.23 With predominant disturbance of other emotions
	.24 With predominant disturbance of conduct
	.25 With mixed disturbance of emotions and conduct
	.28 With other specified predominant symptoms
F43.8	Other reactions to severe stress
F43.9	reaction to severe stress, unspecified

F44   Dissociative (conversion) disorders

F44.0	Dissociative amnesia
F44.1	Dissociative fugue
F44.2	Dissociative stupor
F44.3	Trance and possession disorders#
F44.4	Dissociative motor disorders
F44.5	Dissociative convulsions
F44.6	Dissociative anaesthesia and sensory loss
F44.7	Mixed dissociative (conversion) disorders
F44.8	Other dissociative (conversion) disorders
	.80 Ganser's syndrome
	.81 Multiple personality disorder
	.82 Transient dissociative (conversion) disorders occurring in childhood and adolescence
	.88 Other specified dissociative (conversion) disorders
F44.9	Dissociative (conversion) disorder, unspecified

F45   Somatoform disorders

F45.0	Somatization disorder
F45.1	Undifferentiated somatoform disorder
F45.2	Hypochondrial disorders
F45.3	Somatoform autonomic dysfunction
	.30 Heart and cardiovascular system
	.31 Upper gastrointestinal tract
	.32 Lower gastrointestinal tract
	.33 Respiratory system
	.34 Genitourinary system
	.38 Other organ or system
F45.4	Persistent somatoform pain disorder
F45.8	Other somatoform disorders
F45.9	Somatoform disorder, unspecified

F48   Other neurotic disorders

F48.0	Neurasthenia
F48.1	Depersonalization–derealization syndrome
F48.8	Other specified neurotic disorders
F48.9	Neurotic disorder, unspecified

F50–F59
Behavioural syndromes associated with physiological disturbances and physical factors

F50   Eating disorders

F50.0	Anorexia nervosa
F50.1	Atypical anorexia nervosa
F50.2	Bulimia nervosa
F50.3	Atypical bulimia nervosa
F50.4	Overeating associated with other psychological disturbances
F50.5	Vomiting associated with other psychological disturbances
F50.8	Other eating disorders
F50.9	Eating disorder, unspecified

F51   Non-organic sleep disorders

F51.0	Non-organic insomnia
F51.1	Non-organic hypersomnia
F51.2	Non-organic disorder of the sleep–wake schedule
F51.3	Sleepwalking (somnambulism)
F51.4	Sleep terrors (night terrors)
F51.5	Nightmares
F51.8	Other non-organic sleep disorders
F51.9	Non-organic sleep disorder, unspecified

F52	**Sexual dysfunction, not caused by organic disorder or disease**
F52.0	Lack or loss of sexual desire
F52.1	Sexual aversion and lack of sexual enjoyment
	.10 Sexual aversion
	.11 Lack of sexual enjoyment
F52.2	Failure of genital response
F52.3	Orgasmic dysfunction
F52.4	Premature ejaculation
F52.5	Non-organic vaginismus
F52.6	Non-organic dyspareunia
F52.7	Excessive sexual drive
F52.8	Other sexual dysfunction, not caused by organic disorder or disease
F52.9	Unspecified sexual dysfunction, not caused by organic disorder or disease

F53 **Mental and behavioural disorders associated with the puerperium, not elsewhere classified**

F53.0 Mild mental and behavioural disorders associated with the puerperium, not elsewhere classified

F53.1 Severe mental and behavioural disorders associated with the puerperium, not elsewhere classified

F53.8 Other mental and behavioural disorders associated with the puerperium, not elsewhere classified

F53.9 Puerperal mental disorder, unspecified

F54 **Psychological and behavioural factors associated with disorders or diseases classified elsewhere**

F55 **Abuse of non-dependence-producing substances**

F55.0 Antidepressants
F55.1 Laxatives
F55.2 Analgesics
F55.3 Antacids
F55.4 Vitamins
F55.5 Steroids or hormones
F55.6 Specific herbal or folk remedies
F55.8 Other substances that do not produce dependence
F55.9 Unspecified

F59 **Unspecified behavioural syndromes associated with physiological disturbances and physical factors**

F60–69
Disorders of adult personality and behaviour

F60 **Specific personality disorder**
F60.0 Paranoid personality disorder
F60.1 Schizoid personality disorder
F60.2 Dissocial personality disorder
F60.3 Emotionally unstable personality disorder
    .30 Impulsive type
    .31 Borderline type
F60.4 Histrionic personality disorder
F60.5 Anankastic personality disorder
F60.6 Anxious (avoidant) personality disorder
F60.7 Dependent personality disorder
F60.8 Other specific personality disorder
F60.9 Personality disorder, unspecified

F61 **Mixed and other personality disorders**
F61.0 Mixed personality disorder
F61.1 Troublesome personality changes

F62 **Enduring personality changes, not attributable to brain damage and disease**
F62.0 Enduring personality change after catastrophic experience
F62.1 Enduring personality change after psychiatric illness
F62.8 Other enduring personality changes
F62.9 Enduring personality change, unspecified

F63 **Habit and impulsive disorders**
F63.0 Pathological gambling
F63.1 Pathological fire-setting (pyromania)
F63.2 Pathological stealing (kleptomania)
F63.3 Trichotillomania
F63.8 Other habit and impulsive disorders
F63.8 Habit and impulse disorder, unspecified

F64 **Gender identity disorders**
F64.0 Transsexualism
F64.1 Dual-role transvestism
F64.2 Gender identity disorder of childhood
F64.8 Other gender identity disorders
F64.9 Gender identity disorder, unspecified

F65 **Disorders of sexual preference**
F65.0 Fetishism
F65.1 Fetishistic transvestism
F65.2 Exhibitionism

F65.3	Voyeurism
F65.4	Paedophilia
F65.5	Sadomasochism
F65.6	Multiple disorders of sexual preference
F65.8	Other disorders of sexual preference
F65.9	Disorder of sexual preference, unspecified
F66	Psychological and behavioural disorders associated with sexual development and orientation
F66.0	Sexual maturation disorder
F66.1	Egodystonic sexual orientation
F66.2	Sexual relationship disorder
F66.8	Other psychosexual development disorders
F66.9	Psychosexual development disorder, unspecified

A fifth character may be used to indicate association with:

.x0	Heterosexuality
.x1	Homosexuality
.x2	Bisexuality
.x8	Other, including prepubertal

F68 Other disorder of adult personality and behaviour

F68.0	Elaboration of physical symptoms for psychological reasons
F68.1	Intentional production or feigning of symptoms or disabilities, either physical or psychological (factitious disorder)
F68.8	Other specified disorders of adult personality and behaviour

F69 Unspecified disorder of adult personality and behaviour

F70–F79
Mental retardation

F70 Mild mental retardation

F71 Moderate mental retardation

F72 Severe mental retardation

F73 Profound mental retardation

F78 Other mental retardation

F79 Unspecified mental retardation

A fourth character may be used to specify the extent of associated impairment of behaviour:

F7x.0	No, or minimal, impairment of behaviour
F7x.1	Significant impairment of behaviour requiring
	attention or treatment
F7x.2	Other impairments of behaviour
F7x.3	Without mention of impairment of behaviour

F80–F89
Disorders of psychological development

F80 Specific developmental disorders of speech and language

F80.0	Specific speech articulation disorder
F80.1	Expressive language disorder
F80.2	Receptive language disorder
F80.3	Acquired aphasia with epilepsy (Landau-Kleffner syndrome)
F80.8	Other developmental disorders of speech and language
F80.9	Developmental disorder of speech and language, unspecified

F81 Specific developmental disorders of scholastic skills

F81.0	Specific reading disorder
F81.1	Specific spelling disorder
F81.2	Specific disorder of arithmetical skills
F81.3	Mixed disorder of scholastic skills
F81.8	Other developmental disorders of scholastic skills
F81.9	Developmental disorder of scholastic skills, unspecified

F82 Specific developmental disorder of motor function

F83 Mixed specific developmental disorder

F84 Pervasive developmental disorders

F84.0	Childhood autism
F84.1	Atypical autism
	*.10 Atypicality in age of onset
	*.11 Atypicality in symptomatology
	*.12 Atypicality in both age of onset and symptomatology
F84.2	Rett's syndrome
F84.3	Other childhood disintegrative disorder
F84.4	Overactive disorder associated with mental retardation and stereotyped movements
F84.5	Asperger's syndrome
F84.8	Other pervasive developmental disorders
F84.9	Pervasive developmental disorder, unspecified

F88 Other disorders of psychological development

F89   Unspecified disorder of psychological development

F90–F98
Behavioural and emotional disorders with onset during occurring in childhood and adolescence

F90   Hyperkinetic disorder
F90.0   Disturbance of activity and attention
F90.1   Hyperkinetic conduct disorder
F90.8   Other hyperkinetic disorders
F90.9   Hyperkinetic disorder, unspecified

F91   Conduct disorders
F91.0   Conduct disorder confined to the family context
F92.2   Socialized conduct disorder
F92.3   Oppositional defiant disorder
F92.8   Other conduct disorders
F92.9   Conduct disorder, unspecified

F92   Mixed disorders of conduct and emotions
F92.0   Depressive conduct disorder
F92.8   Other mixed disorders of conduct and emotions
F92.9   Mixed disorder of conduct and emotions, unspecified

F93   Emotional disorders with onset specific to childhood
F93.0   Separation anxiety disorder of childhood
F93.1   Phobic anxiety disorder of childhood
F93.2   Social anxiety disorder of childhood
F93.3   Sibling rivalry disorder
F93.8   Other childhood emotional disorders
         *.80 Generalized anxiety disorder of childhood
F93.9   Childhood emotional disorder, unspecified

F94   Disorders of social functioning with onset specific to childhood and adolescence
F94.0   Elective mutism
F94.1   Reactive attachment disorder of childhood
F94.2   Disinhibited attachment disorder of childhood
F94.8   Other childhood disorders of social functioning

F94.9   Childhood disorder of social functioning, unspecified

F95   Tic disorders
F95.0   Transient tic disorders
F95.1   Chronic motor or vocal tic disorder
F95.2   Combined vocal and multiple motor tic disorder (de la Tourette's syndrome)
F95.8   Other tic disorders
F95.9   Tic disorder, unspecified

F98   Other behavioural and emotional disorders with onset usually occurring in childhood and adolescence
F98.0   Non-organic enuresis
         *.00 Nocturnal enuresis only
         *.01 Diurnal enuresis only
         *.02 Nocturnal and diurnal enureses
F98.1   Non-organic encopresis
         *.10 Failure to acquire physiological bowel control
         *.11 Adequate bowel control with normal faeces deposited in inappropriate places
         *.12 Soiling that is associated with excessively fluid faeces, such as with retention with overflow
F98.2   Feeding disorder of infancy and childhood
F98.3   Pica of infancy and childhood
F98.4   Stereotyped movement disorders
         *.40 Non-self-injurious
         *.41 Self-injurious
         *.42 Mixed
F98.5   Stuttering (stammering)
F98.6   Cluttering
F98.8   Other specified behavioural and emotional disorders with onset usually occurring in childhood and adolescence
F98.9   Unspecified behavioural and emotional disorders with onset usually occurring in childhood and adolescence

F99
Unspecified mental disorder

F99   Mental disorder, not otherwise specified

Appendix B

Languages into which the ICD-10 Classification of Mental Disorders Clinical Descriptions and Diagnostic Guidelines and Diagnostic Criteria for Research have been translated:

1. CDDG

Language	Publisher	Year
Chinese	People's Medical Publishing House, Beijing	1993
Czech	Czech Psychiatric Association, Prague	1992
Danish	Munksgaard, Copenhagen (short glossary only)	1994
Dutch	Swets & Zeitlinger B.V., Lisse	1994
Estonian	Tartu Ulikooli psuhhiaatria keteeder, Tartu	1993
French	Masson Editeur, Paris	1993
German	Verlag Hans Huber, Bern	1991
Greek	Beta Medical Publishers Ltd, Athens	1993
Indonesian	Directorate of Mental Health, Ministry of Health, Djakarta	1993
Italian	Masson Spa, Milan	1992
Japanese	Igaku-Shoin Ltd, Tokyo	1993
Korean	Il Cho Kak Publishers, Seoul	1994
Portuguese	Editora Artes Médicas Sul Ltda, Porto Algre	1993
Russian	Hippocrates Publishing House, St Petersburg	1994
Serbian	Zavod za Idzbenike i Nastavna Sredstva, Belgrade	1992
Spanish	Meditor, Madrid	1992
Thai	Mental Health Division, Ministry of Public Health, Bangkok	1993
Turkish	Turkish Society for Mental & Neurological Health, Hacettepe Universitesi, Ankara	1992
Vietnamese	Trung uong, Hanoi	1992

2. DCR

Dutch	Swets & Zeitlinger B.V., Lisse	1994
French	Masson, Paris	1994
German	Clausen & Bosse, Leck	1994
Italian	Masson Spa, Milan	1995
Japanese	Igaku-Shoin Ltd, Tokyo	1994
Russian	Hippocrates, St Petersburg	1994
Spanish	Meditor, Madrid	1994

Appendix C

WHO REFERENCE AND TRAINING CENTRES ON CLASSIFICATION, DIAGNOSIS AND ASSESSMENT OF MENTAL AND BEHAVIOURAL DISORDER

China	Professor Shen Yucun Institute of Mental Health Beijing Medical University Beijing 100083 People's Republic of China Tel: (00861) 209 1953 or 202 7314 Fax: (00861) 202 7314	Chinese
Denmark	Dr A. Bertelsen Institute of Psychiatric Demography Psychiatric Hospital University of Aarhus 8240 Risskov, Denmark Tel: +45 (86) 17 77 77 Fax: +45 (86) 17 59 77	Danish
Egypt	Dr A. Okasha Department of Psychiatry Ain Shams University 3 Shawarby Street Kasr-El-Nil Cairo, Egypt Tel: +20 (2) 710 233 Fax: +20 (2) 348 1786	Arabic
Germany	Dr H. Dilling Klinik fur Psychiatrie der Medizinischen Hochschule Ratzeburger Allee 160 23562 Lubeck Germany Tel: +49 (451) 500 2440 Fax: +49 (451) 500 2603	German
India	Dr R.S. Murthy National Institute of Mental Health & Neurosciences Kannada Department of Psychiatry Bangalore 560029 India Tel: +91 (80) 6652121 Fax: +91 (80) 6431830	Hindi

Japan	Dr Y. Nakane	Japanese
	Department of Neuropsychiatry	
	Nagasaki University, School of Medicine	
	7-1 Sakamoto-Machi	
	Nagasaki 852, Japan	
	Tel: +81 (958) 47 21 11	
	Fax: +81 (958) 49 43 72	

Japan   Dr Y. Nakane   Japanese
                        Department of Neuropsychiatry
                        Nagasaki University, School of Medicine
                        7-1 Sakamoto-Machi
                        Nagasaki 852, Japan
                        Tel: +81 (958) 47 21 11
                        Fax: +81 (958) 49 43 72

Luxembourg   Dr Ch. Pull   French
                        Service de Neuropsychiatrie
                        Centre Hospitalier de Luxembourg
                        4 rue Barble
                        1210 Luxembourg
                        Tel: +352 4411 2256
                        Fax: +352 458 762

Spain   Dr J.J. Lopez   Spanish
                        Servicio de Psiquiatria
                        Hospital Universitario San Carlos
                        28040 Madrid
                        Spain
                        Tel/fax: +34 (1) 330 3574

United Kingdom   Dr M. Gelder   English
                        Department of Psychiatry
                        Oxford University Hospital
                        Warneford Hospital
                        Old Road, Headington
                        Oxford OX3 7JX
                        United Kingdom
                        Tel: +44 (865) 226 460
                        Fax: +44 (864) 793 101

United States   Dr D. Reiger   English
                        Division of Epidemiology & Services
                        Research
                        NIMH, Room 10-105
                        5600 Fishers Lane
                        Rockville, MD 20857, USA
                        Tel: +1 (301) 443 3648
                        Fax: +1 (301) 443 4045